THE PROTEIN LIFESTYLE

THE PROTEIN LIFESTYLE
COOKBOOK

A Guide to Cooking Delicious and
Easy-to-Prepare, High-Protein Recipies

Joshua D. Noland
JoshNoland.com

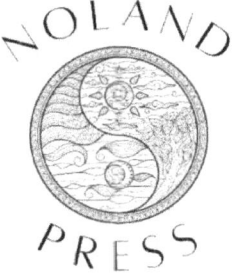

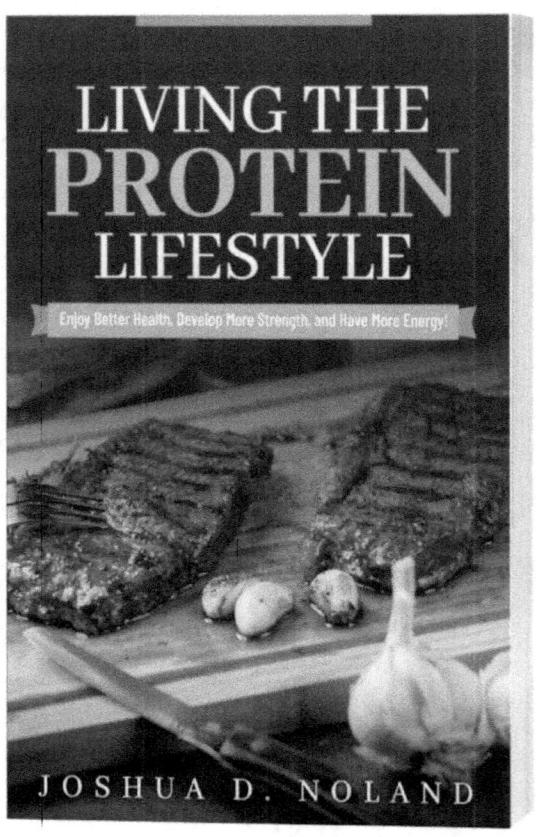

Living The Protein Lifestyle is the groundbreaking first book in the Protein Lifestyle series, chronicling Joshua D. Noland's extraordinary health evolution. Discover how Joshua conquered depression, broke free from food addiction, and lost over eighty pounds. This book includes powerful strategies and transformative techniques to help you unlock your best self—inside and out. Joshua's holistic approach goes beyond protein, incorporating mental wellness and staying active for a complete lifestyle upgrade. Learn how to create sustainable change with easy-to-implement steps that empower you to reclaim your health and vitality. Whether you're looking to build strength, boost energy, or cultivate peace of mind, *Living The Protein Lifestyle* will inspire you to take control and thrive.

ProteinLifestyleBook.com

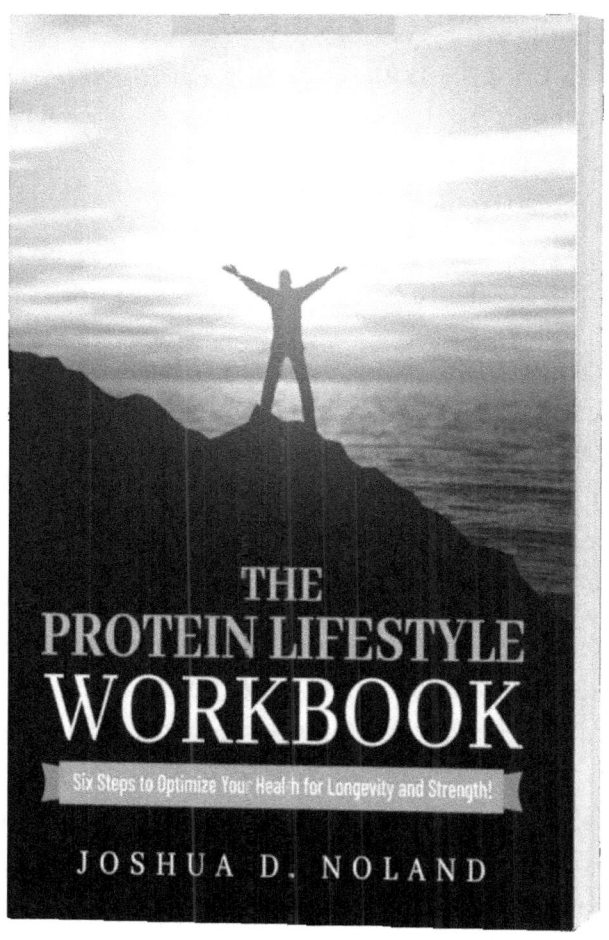

THE
PROTEIN LIFESTYLE
WORKBOOK

Six Steps to Optimize Your Health for Longevity and Strength!

JOSHUA D. NOLAND

Are you prepared to unlock your full potential? Do you need a clear, actionable guide to transform your health? This revolutionary workbook, *The Protein Lifestyle Workbook,* is the second book in the Protein Lifestyle series. It provides a step-by-step blueprint designed to help you achieve lasting health success. With crystal-clear guidance and easy-to-follow steps, you'll take confident action toward creating the vibrant, energized life you deserve—at your own pace. Whether starting fresh or looking to elevate your current routine, this workbook empowers you to make impactful, sustainable changes that fit seamlessly into your lifestyle.

ProteinLifestyleWorkbook.com

The Protein Lifestyle Cookbook
A Guide to Cooking Delicious and Easy-to-Prepare, High-Protein Recipes
By Joshua D. Noland
Copyright © 2024 Joshua D. Noland

ISBN: 978-1-965040-02-7

The information in this cookbook should not be treated as a substitute for professional medical or clinical advice; always consult a medical or clinical practitioner. Any use of information in this cookbook is at the reader's discretion and risk. Neither the author nor the publisher can be held responsible for any loss, claim, or damage arising from the use or misuse of the suggestions made, the failure to take medical or clinical advice, or for any material on third-party websites.

If you have any food allergies, dietary restrictions, or health conditions, consult a medical professional or registered dietitian before consuming any recipes in this book. Additionally, the author and publisher shall not be held responsible for any kitchen mishaps, equipment failures, or adverse reactions from preparing or consuming recipes in this cookbook.

Preparing and handling raw ingredients, particularly meats, seafood, and eggs, require caution to prevent foodborne illness. Please ensure proper hygiene and cooking techniques to minimize risk.

WHY THIS COOKBOOK

Are you tired of feeling sick and tired? Do you want to discover low-carb, high-protein recipes that actually taste good and nourish your body so you can look and feel your best? This cookbook is exactly what you've been looking for. I have spent years perfecting these recipes, and I can assure you that they taste great, will nourish your body, and satisfy your hunger throughout the day. This cookbook is the key to unlocking lasting health success.

Let food be thy medicine, and let medicine be thy food.

*— **Hippocrates***

I Lost over Eighty Pounds and Overcame IBS, Depression, and Food Addiction by Eating These Foods

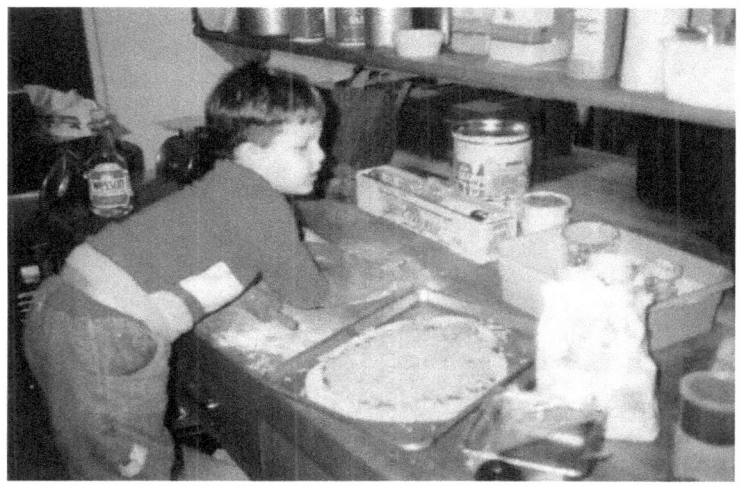

Joshua D. Noland is a chef and health advocate. He has studied nutrition and health at Stanford University and his real-world experience in the food service industry has given him extensive inside knowledge of how to improve the nutrient profile of food without sacrificing flavor. His passion is helping others develop healthy habits to improve their quality of life and live intentionally. He advocates for regenerative agriculture, whole foods, an active lifestyle, and emphasizes the significance of mental well-being for overall health. He was able to take control of his health by following the protein lifestyle and has found lasting success. Visit JoshNoland.com to learn more about him and take advantage of his free resources.

Table of Contents

"If you only prioritize protein, you'll feel better, get stronger, and live longer."

"The only real stumbling block is fear of failure. In cooking, you've got to have a what-the-hell attitude."

— Julia Child

EGGSPERT

Do you know how to make scrambled eggs?

They're one of the simplest things to make, but countless variations exist. Whether you're an eggspert or new to cooking, you can prepare these recipes and learn new innovative techniques in this cookbook.

Cooking is one of the most valuable skills to learn. If you know how to prepare food, you will never go hungry or be forced to buy prepackaged foods that may harm your health. It doesn't take long to get the hang of it either, and it's never too late to learn how to make good food that will fuel your body and satisfy your taste buds. Once you learn a few basic cooking techniques, you can make a wide variety of dishes. I have included a chapter on basic cooking skills and another on basic cooking methods to help you feel more confident in the kitchen.

Anyone can learn to cook, and cooking with others is a great way to bond and learn new skills and techniques. Sharing a meal you cooked together will bring you closer and can be fun. We are social creatures, and eating together is an integral part of our social structure.

The Protein Lifestyle is a way of life that leads to health and happiness. This cookbook is the third book in the Protein Lifestyle series. The first book in the series, *Living the Protein Lifestyle,* is where I share my health evolution story. It includes how I lost over seventy pounds and overcame food addiction and depression. I share the proven strategies and methods I was able to incorporate into my life to find lasting success. The second is *The Protein Lifestyle Workbook*, a step-by-step guide designed to help develop a lifestyle that increases your health over time and allows you to enjoy the foods you love. This cookbook was created to teach you how to cook those foods that will satiate your hunger, satisfy your taste buds, nourish your body, and help you hit your daily protein goals.

The recipes are primarily animal-based because these foods offer a complete amino acid profile in the exact quantities and ratios our bodies need to function at their best. Vegetables don't have enough protein or the right kind, so if you're a vegan or vegetarian, these recipes are not for you.

Everyone is different and there's not one diet that's right for everyone. Some may need more carbohydrates, especially for women during specific menstrual cycles, so determine what's best for your body and do that.

Protein is the most underrated and under-consumed health food on the planet. That's why it's the main attraction in most of these recipes. You should eat about one gram of protein per pound of your ideal body weight daily. That is just a general rule, as some may need more or less depending on multiple factors, but most people consume well short of this general rule and could benefit significantly by adding more meat to their diet.

While we are on the subject of nutrition, I need to say I have realized that if you want to lose weight, you have to limit the amount of carbohydrates you eat. Fat and carbohydrates are both excellent energy sources, but if you are using carbs as energy, you are not burning fat.

Something else to consider is when you combine salt, fat, and carbs together, they trigger a natural urge to gorge. This is an ancient survival method our bodies use to take advantage of times of plenty to get us through times of famine. You don't have to worry about that since food is so abundant in the present day. If you eat carbohydrates, you should isolate fats to reduce the total calories you consume and vice versa.

You can use low-fat dairy products like cottage cheese, Greek yogurt, shredded cheese, egg whites, and lean meats. However, whole-fat foods will provide more nutrients and essential fats. Remember, there are no essential carbohydrates.

I love red meat, and most cuts are naturally fatty, so I tend to stay away from carbohydrates, which is reflected in the recipes.

Fat is critical for many bodily functions and got a bad wrap in the nineteen sixties when the sugar industry-funded research that downplayed the link between sugar and coronary heart disease and shifted the blame to fat, which has influenced public health policies and dietary guidelines for the past few decades. Don't fear dietary fat; it fuels your body and supports your overall health.

Regarding cooking fats, I strongly advise you never to use the processed seed oils that are so prevalent in processed foods and use at most restaurants. These oils are highly inflammatory and oxidize very easily, causing harm to your body.

Stick with less refined fats for cooking, like tallow, lard, butter, extra virgin olive oil, or coconut oil. These fats are minimally processed and can contribute additional nutrients to your diet.

Get ready to discover the recipes that you'll be excited to eat, won't take all day to make or require a culinary degree. I have developed these recipes over many years to make them simple so you can enjoy home-cooked meals even if you don't have much time to devote to cooking. These recipes have been optimized to fuel your body with the nutrients it needs to thrive and satiate your hunger. This is not a diet cookbook. However, these recipes will keep you full, making you less likely to snack in between meals. The recipes focus on using whole food ingredients, appropriate amounts of protein for proper nutrition, and are low in carbohydrates. By eating this way, you will lose weight, overcome chronic disease, and feel good.

The recipes within have helped many people overcome their health struggles, including myself and my father. He was able to beat the threat of diabetes by eating the very foods that you are about to learn how to prepare in this cookbook.

This cookbook will teach you how to cook high-protein meals using whole-food ingredients and how to substitute any ingredients you don't like or don't have on hand.

Discover Additional Recipes, Cooking Tips, and Many More Resources at JoshNoland.com or Use This QR Code:

ABOUT THIS COOKBOOK

I created this carefully curated collection of recipes to help you feel and look your best. Most recipes do not provide enough protein and go overboard on carbohydrates. When you eat more protein and fat, your body is nourished so it can function correctly. I am very passionate about health and genuinely believe in Hippocrates's quote. When you eat the right foods, they provide everything the body needs, and when you combine this with some physical activity, it can help you lose weight and overcome common diseases.

All ingredients are protein lifestyle recommended, but feel free to substitute them for your particular needs.

I have included chapters on basic cooking skills and cooking methods to guide those new to cooking. If that is you, don't be intimidated. You'll be successful in making these recipes and be able to share them with people you love.

This is the protein lifestyle cookbook, and that's the inspiration for how the recipes are organized. Each chapter is organized by the protein featured in each recipe. This way, you can peruse the recipes based on what you have on hand or your preferred proteins.

The recipes have been formatted in a simple and easy-to-read layout, including the nutritional facts to ensure you get enough fat and protein. I also offer variations and substitutions for each dish so you can customize them to your preferences.

I don't have time to cook. If this is what you're thinking, say less. I got you. I have designed most of these recipes to be simple and easy to make but still pack tons of flavor. I have ranked every recipe in this cookbook using my patented meatball difficulty rating. One out of five meatball recipes are the easiest, and five out of five meatball recipes are the most difficult. Common home cooks with standard home cooking equipment can make even the most difficult recipes in this cookbook. They may take more time and include more steps, but you will succeed if you break them down and prepare them in stages.

Cooking good food is a skill that must be practiced to be perfected. Some spend a lifetime experimenting to make the most incredible flavor and texture combinations. Feeding yourself and your loved ones food that tastes good and has healing effects is not hard; you can do this.

Luckily, the protein lifestyle cookbook is here to help you learn how to save time in the kitchen and make food that will improve your longevity and strength! As long as you follow the steps in each recipe and take the time to find high-quality ingredients, you will successfully prepare amazingly delicious meals that will fuel your physical and mental health.

BASIC COOKING SKILLS

If you are a professional cook, you can skip this chapter. If you're not a professional cook or need a refresher on skills like ingredient preparation and time management, read on.

Knife Skills

Knowing how to handle a knife in the kitchen properly will make or break a home cook. If you have basic knife skills, you can save a lot of money by cutting down primal cuts of meat. That is why I will teach you how to use a knife safely and effectively. It may seem counterintuitive, but the sharper the blade, the less likely you are to cut yourself if you are using the proper technique. If your knife is dull, you must use more force, putting yourself at risk.

Hold the knife in your dominant hand and use your other hand to stabilize the item you're cutting. Curl the fingers and thumb of your non-dominant hand so that your fingernails face the blade of the knife as you cut. If your hand gets too close, you'll stop cutting once the blade hits your nail, not your skin.

The closer your hand is to where you are cutting, the more control you will have, so you must find the right balance between being close and not too close. As you cut the item, continually slide your non-dominant hand away from the blade, continuing to use your fingernails as a shield.

Many kinds of kitchen knives exist, but a chef's knife will do for most applications. A few other basic cutting implements that can be very useful in the kitchen include kitchen shears, a paring knife, and a bread or utility knife.

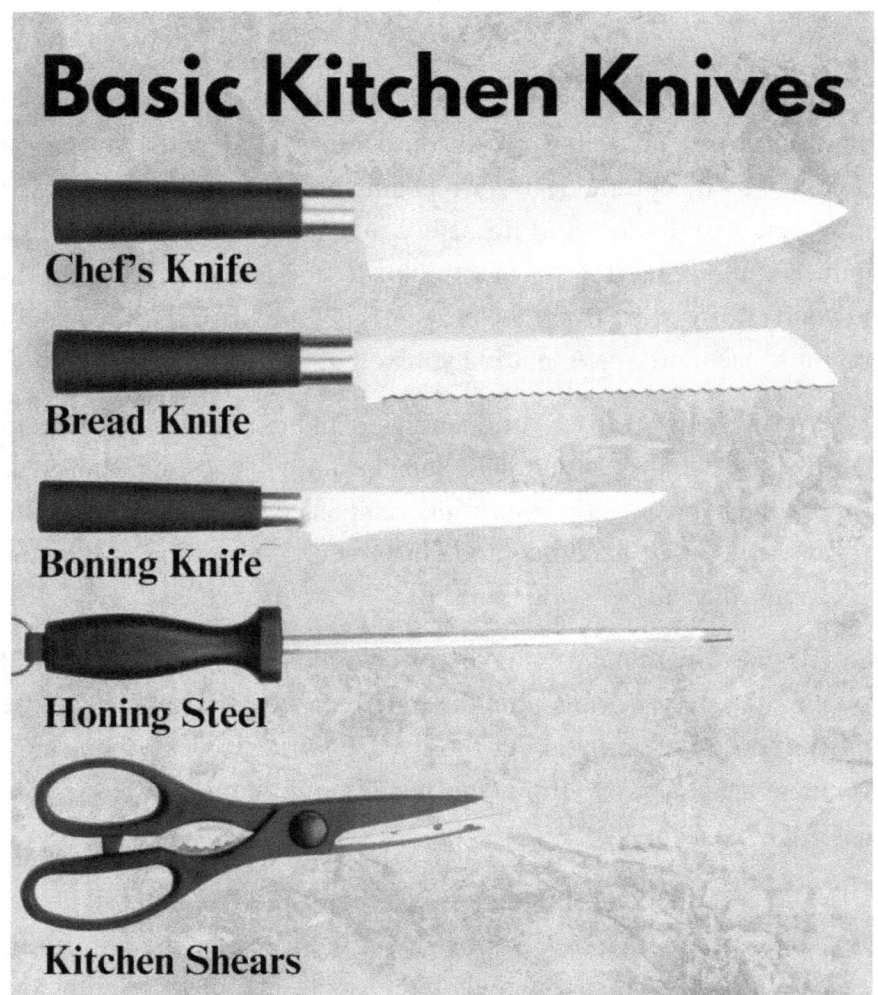

You can use a honing steel to keep your knives tuned up, but only a sharpening stone or another sharpening device will sharpen an already dulled blade. I usually use a handheld sharpener along with a honing steel.

The handheld sharpener is easy to use and is used to sharpen the blade every few months. Place a handheld sharpener on the counter. Use one hand to hold the sharpener firmly on the counter, hold the knife in the other hand, and drag the blade along the grinding surface of the sharpener a few times. Now, you'll only need to use the honing steel to realign the edge to maintain the blade of your sharpened knife once a week or so, depending on how much you use it.

I do this for ease of use, but about once a year, I like to use a sharpening stone to get all my knives very sharp.

Recipes call for many different sizes and shapes of foods, which we call cutting techniques. Some of them are chopped, diced, minced. shredded, and graded. Each technique has its own uses and methods.

Each technique requires a different approach and skill level, from more casual chopping to precise dicing and very fine mincing. These are foundational skills in cooking that can significantly impact your results.

Pro Tip: To prevent your cutting board from slipping, place a wet towel or a piece of shelf liner under it.

Heat Control

Controlling temperatures during cooking is crucial for achieving desired textures and flavors and avoiding over or undercooking foods. We've come a long way from cooking over the raw flames of a campfire, but we still enjoy grilling over open flames. We have more heating options now, so let's discuss how and when to use them.

How to use different heat levels on a stovetop:

High Heat

When to Use:

- Searing Meat: High heat creates a delicious brown crust on meats due to the Maillard reaction.

- Boiling Water: Whether you're making pasta or blanching vegetables, high heat gets the job done quickly.

- Stir-frying: This quick-cooking technique requires high heat to cook vegetables and meats evenly and rapidly.

Tips for Using High Heat:

- Always preheat the pan before adding oil, then preheat the oil before adding the ingredients to ensure even cooking.

- Keep an eye on it; food can go from perfectly browned to burnt in seconds.

Medium Heat

When to Use:

- Sautéing: This method is perfect for cooking vegetables or frying onions until translucent. Medium heat allows for even cooking without burning.

- Cooking Eggs: Delicate items like eggs need a balance of heat to cook through without burning the exterior.

- Simmering Sauces: After boiling a sauce, reducing it to a simmer (a state just below boiling) helps flavors meld together without the risk of burning.

Tips for Using Medium Heat:

- Give your pan some time to reach the desired temperature. When the pan is ready, a water droplet should sizzle—not evaporate immediately or sit still.

- Adjust the heat slightly up or down as needed to maintain a steady simmer or to prevent browning too quickly.

Low Heat

When to Use:

- Melting butter: Low heat ensures that the butter melts evenly without burning.

- Cooking Delicate Fish: Gentle, slow cooking preserves the fish's texture and moisture.

- Braising: Slow cooking at low heat breaks down the tough fibers in meat, making it tender and flavorful.

Tips for Using Low Heat:

- Use a heavy-bottomed pot or pan to distribute the heat evenly and prevent hot spots.

- Patience is key. Low and slow cooking develops deep flavors and textures that can't be achieved with high heat.

You may need to adjust temperatures during cooking to control heat effectively. It often comes down to knowing your equipment, understanding the ingredients you're working with, and keeping a close eye on the process. Try to be flexible. You don't have to follow the recipe exactly unless you're baking. Adjust the heat as needed. If ingredients are browning too quickly, reduce the heat. If you are trying to boil something and it turns into a simmer, simply increase the heat.

In general, you'll want to start cooking most dishes on high heat and then finish on low heat. Starting on high to sear or boil and then reducing to low heat for a simmer or braise allows for both flavor development and tenderness in the final dish.

Residual heat is another important aspect of cooking. Even after you turn off the flame, your dish will continue cooking due to the residual heat. This is from the residual heat in the pan and the burner. For example, after sautéing vegetables, you might remove them from the heat a few minutes before they reach the desired doneness, letting the residual heat finish the job.

Practice and attention will improve your ability to judge when and how to adjust the heat properly.

Ingredient Preparation

Before you start cooking, you must have all your ingredients ready. This includes washing, peeling, cutting, and measuring. One of the best takeaways from my time in culinary school is the French term mise en place *"meez ahn plahs."* This translates to everything in its place. This method of preparing everything and having it ready and available makes cooking more enjoyable and ensures you have everything you need before you get going, and timing becomes crucial.

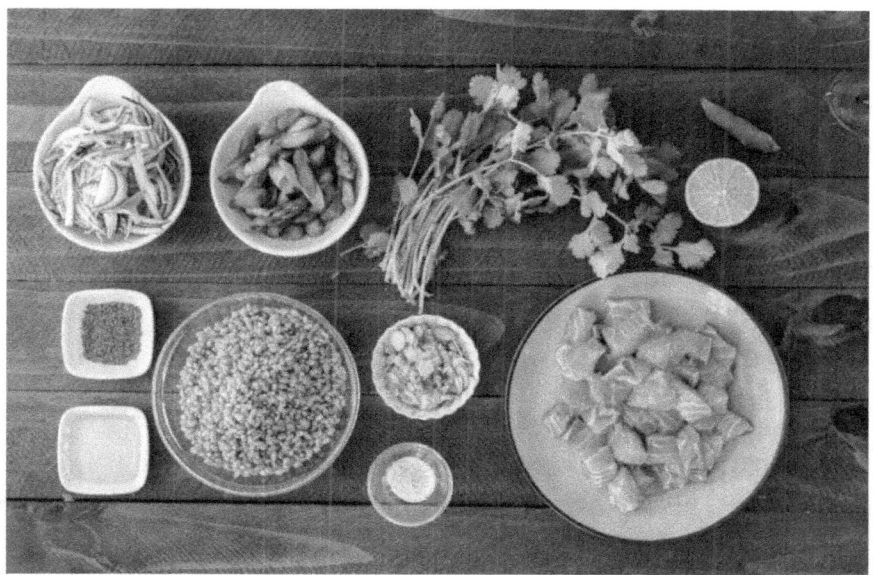

To do this right, you will need some small deli containers or bowls to put the prepared and premeasured ingredients. This will help you stay organized and keep track of what you've already done.

Consider this scenario:

You're making meatball casserole and are right in the middle of adding the seasonings when someone knocks on your door. You stop what you're doing, answer the door, and when you get back, you forget what you've already added.

If you had been practicing mise en place, you would see the containers of ingredients you have or haven't added and know where you left off.

This becomes more critical when you start sautéing onions and don't have the next ingredient ready, and your onions start to burn.

Mise en place is excellent for ensuring you have everything you need when you start cooking, but taking measures to avoid food-borne illnesses is another part of ingredient preparation.

You must thoroughly wash all produce to remove dirt and harmful chemical residues. Cross-contamination from raw meat is also a valid concern, so when working with it, make sure to wash your hands, cutting board, and any other surface that may have come into contact with raw meat.

When pealing, trimming, or any other prep that involves removing inedible parts of foods, keep a bowl on the counter next to you to put the waist in. This will save you time going back and forth to the trash can.

Understanding Flavors

Making food taste good is strange when you stop to think about it. We naturally crave certain flavors due to how we evolved on this planet to get the proper nutrients we need to fuel, grow, and maintain our bodies, but in the last one hundred years or so, people have been developing foods that highjack our natural cravings and make it very hard for us to eat instinctively.

The Dorito Effect by Mark Schatzker goes into this phenomenon in great detail. Basically, all of the artificial and "natural" flavorings added to ultra-processed food products have killed our intuitive eating abilities, so we associate chemicals with nutrition. It used to be that when our bodies needed a specific nutrient, we would crave that food, but now, foods are so fake that our bodies have mostly lost that ability. Only when we abstain from eating these highly engineered food products can our bodies regain their ability to tell us what nutrients we need again. It's not easy, this shit is everywhere, and it's highly addicting.

Seeking flavor is not inherently wrong but can be a slippery slope. We should be eating to fuel our bodies, but some foods taste so good it's hard to eat the foods our bodies require to function at their best. Lucky for you, I have developed the recipes in this cookbook to satisfy your taste buds and nutritional needs.

You can make food that tastes good and is good for you. If a certain recipe calls for water, replace it with broth, milk, or another ingredient that fits the dish. You want to add flavor wherever possible to make a dish with a complex flavor profile that you and your loved ones will want to eat.

If you make healthy food that does not taste good, you won't look forward to eating it and may stray from good eating habits. You should be enjoying life to its fullest potential. You eat three times a day, which is sixty to ninety meals a month. If you want to live your life to the fullest, you need to be able to eat food that you love and will love you back.

One of the best parts about cooking is you can customize each dish to suit your preferences. Whatever you do, make each dish your own by adding and substituting whatever you need to make it yours.

Time Management

Cooking is all about time management. You'll want all of the components of a dish to be at the optimal temperature when you serve them, and this can present unique challenges when you are serving multiple items to make a complete meal.

This process is manageable with some foresight and planning. Luckily, most of the recipes in this cookbook are designed with this in mind, and they will taste the best immediately after being cooked.

Strangely enough, some recipes, like my teriyaki chicken fried rice, are better the next day. It has to do with the flavors all melding together after the dish cools down. Either way, when planning meals, read the entire recipe in advance to ensure you have all of the necessary ingredients and be familiar with the steps involved. Some recipes will have steps that require things to marinate overnight or have steps that can be split up over a day or so to make the final preparation smoother. This can be achieved by preparing ingredients in advance and having them ready to go when you are ready to complete the dish.

Coordinating and managing cooking times is crucial for simultaneously preparing multiple components of a meal. Understanding when to start each element of a dish to ensure everything is ready at the same time is a vital skill.

Weighing Ingredients

This is not a cooking skill per se, but it is cooking adjacent. Being able to use a digital kitchen scale can save you time when measuring out ingredients and cleaning. Consider using just one bowl to weigh all your ingredients using the tare function on your digital scale. The tare function returns the weight to zero even if something is on the scale, like a bowl. This can come in very handy as you can put your bowl on the scale, zero out the weight, and then start adding ingredients—for example, my blender ice cream recipe. Place the blender pitcher on the scale, tap tare, weigh your frozen fruit of choice, then blend it. Place the pitcher back on the scale, tap the tare button, add the cream, blend it, and enjoy. This way, you only have to wash the blender pitcher and a rubber spatula.

Pro tip: Place your scale on a flat, level surface for accurate measurement.

Using a scale to weigh cooked meat is another fantastic use of this vital kitchen tool. When you weigh your protein versus measuring by volume or eyeballing it, you will have a much more accurate account of how much protein you consume, which can make a big difference over time.

Chapter summary:

If you are missing an ingredient, it's okay. You can always substitute or leave it out entirely, depending on the recipe and what you are missing. Don't sweat it if you don't have parsley for your chicken soup. Your chicken soup will still taste great without it. Don't let little bumps in the road, like not having one ingredient, get in your way. Use what you have and make it work. This is what Julia Childs meant when she said, "You've got to have a what-the-hell attitude."

Now that you know some basic cooking skills, put them to the test and cook something amazing today.

"Cooking is an observation-based process that you can't do if you're so completely focused on a recipe."

— Alton Brown

COOKING METHODS

In this chapter, I discuss the basic cooking methods called for in the recipes throughout the cookbook so you can be more familiar with them and learn how they differ from each other.

Air Frying

Air frying has become a healthier alternative to deep frying in recent years. It's similar to convection baking but uses more concentrated heat and faster airflow to make your food crispy. It uses less oil, resulting in faster cooking time and less cleanup. I love air frying, and I use it a lot; it's convenient and speeds up cooking time. They are not suitable for all applications, but when they are, they work great. When frying bacon, The grease falls down to the base of the basket, and the crispy bacon produced is superb.

There are different types of air fryers, and they do not all cook the same. Toaster oven-style air fryers are great and can do way more than just air frying, but they can not compare with basket-style air fryers. The way the basket-style air fryers are set up, with the heating element directly above the food and the fan blowing that heat down onto it, makes it cook hotter and quicker. The downside is that you must cook in small batches, or your food won't crisp up.

I have both of these air fryers and use them for different applications. I like the toaster oven style for making bigger dishes and finishing off with the broiler, and I like the basket style for bacon, as I mentioned.

Some people are skeptical of these newer devices, but that's normal with new things. I love air fryers and highly recommend them. The only thing you need to be careful of is that many of them use toxic nonstick coatings on the baskets, so make sure to get one that does not.

Boiling

Boiling is a fundamental cooking method that involves heating liquids to their boiling point. This straightforward technique is versatile and widely used in home kitchens to prepare various foods, including rice, potatoes, and eggs. Boiling is also used to make stocks, soups, and stews, where prolonged exposure to heat helps extract flavors from ingredients.

Braising

Braising is a cooking technique that combines both dry and wet heat to produce tender, flavorful dishes. It involves first searing the food, typically meat or vegetables, at a high temperature to develop a rich, caramelized exterior and then cooking it slowly in a covered pot with a small amount of liquid, such as broth. This method is especially effective for tougher cuts of meat like chuck roast, as the prolonged cooking time at a low temperature breaks down the collagen and connective tissues, resulting in a tender, succulent final product.

Broiling

Broiling is a high-heat cooking method that uses direct radiant heat from an overhead source, typically within an oven. This technique is excellent for quickly cooking or finishing foods like meats, fish, vegetables, and even certain fruits. The intense heat caramelizes the exterior of the food, creating a crispy, flavorful crust while keeping the interior moist and tender.

Pan-Frying

Pan-frying is a cooking method that involves cooking food in a small amount of oil or fat in a shallow pan over medium to high heat.

This technique is perfect for achieving a crispy, golden-brown exterior while keeping the inside moist and flavorful. Pan-frying is commonly used for various foods, including meats and vegetables. I highly recommend using beef tallow or any other animal fat for pan-frying, as ultra-processed seed oils like corn, soy, and canola have been proven to oxidize in the body, causing inflammation and leading to a slew of chronic diseases.

Grilling

Grilling is a cooking method that involves cooking food over direct heat to create a distinctive smoky flavor and a crispy exterior while keeping the interior juicy and tender. This technique has ancient roots, dating back to early humans who cooked food over open fires. Over time, grilling has evolved with the development of various types of grills and fuels, becoming a popular cooking method worldwide.

There are several types of grills that home cooks can choose from, each offering unique benefits:

Gas Grills:

These grills use propane or natural gas as fuel, providing convenience. They are easy to light and offer precise temperature control. Gas grills are ideal for quick grilling sessions and minimal cleanup, making them a popular choice for everyday use.

Charcoal Grills:

Known for producing high heat and a classic smoky flavor, charcoal grills use charcoal briquettes or lump charcoal as fuel. While they require more time and effort to light and manage temperature, many grilling enthusiasts prefer the rich flavor that charcoal grilling imparts. I prefer and recommend using mesquite lump charcoal as it burns very hot and adds a wonderfully earthy, bold flavor to your dish.

Wood Grills:

Using hardwoods like oak, hickory, or mesquite, wood grills offer an authentic smoky flavor. They require significant skill to manage the fire and temperature, but they are favored by purists who appreciate the deep, rich flavors they produce.

Grilling techniques and flavors vary widely across cultures. American barbecue, Argentine asado, and Japanese yakitori are just a few examples of how different regions have developed unique grilling traditions. Each method offers distinct flavors and cooking styles, showcasing the versatility of grilling as a cooking method.

For home cooks looking to enhance their grilling experience, it is important to preheat the grill, clean the grates, use a meat thermometer, experiment with marinades and rubs, and allow the meat to rest after grilling. By mastering these tips and understanding the different types of grills, you can create delicious, restaurant-quality dishes in your own backyard for a fraction of the price.

Pressure Cooking

The Instant Pot is a game-changer in the kitchen, combining multiple cooking methods into one handy appliance. It's not just a pressure cooker; it can also slow cook, sauté, steam, and more. This versatility makes it a must-have for home cooks looking to save time and effort without sacrificing flavor.

One of the standout features of the Instant Pot is its ability to pressure cook. Pressure cooking takes the slow cooking concept and kicks it up a notch. Increasing the pressure inside the pot actually lowers the water's boiling point. This means your food cooks much faster than traditional methods, yet you still get those tender, flavorful results you'd expect from hours of slow cooking. Imagine making a pot roast that falls apart with a fork in under an hour instead of all day—it's a real time-saver!

But that's just the beginning. The Instant Pot can also function as a slow cooker, perfect for those days when you want to set it and forget it. It's great for making chili, stews, and even yogurt. And let's not forget the sauté function, which allows you to brown meat or sauté veggies right in the pot before switching to another cooking mode. This means fewer dishes to wash and more flavor in your meals.

Poaching

Poaching is a gentle cooking method that simmers food in a liquid at a relatively low temperature, typically between 160°F and 180°F. Unlike boiling, which can be too harsh for delicate foods like eggs, poaching allows for slow, even cooking, resulting in tender, flavorful dishes.

Roasting

Roasting is a dry-heat cooking method that involves cooking food in an oven at a high temperature, typically between 375°F and 450°F. The oven's hot air cooks the food evenly on all sides, creating a caramelized, crispy exterior while keeping the inside juicy and tender.

Sautéing

Sautéing is a quick and efficient cooking method that involves cooking food in a small amount of oil or fat over high heat in a shallow pan. The word "sauté" comes from the French word for "jump," reflecting how food is often tossed or stirred in the pan to ensure even cooking. This technique is perfect for browning and caramelizing food, creating a delicious, flavorful crust while keeping the interior moist and tender.

Carbon steel and cast iron skillets are excellent choices when it comes to choosing the right pan for sautéing, unlike non-stick cookware, which can contain toxic chemicals like PFOA and PFTE that may leach into food at high temperatures and cause harm to your body. Carbon steel and cast iron cookware is free from these chemicals. They also offer superior heat distribution and retention, essential for achieving a perfect sauté.

Carbon steel skillets are lightweight and heat up quickly, making them ideal for rapid cooking. With proper seasoning, they also develop a natural non-stick surface over time. Cast iron skillets provide excellent heat retention and can go from stovetop to oven, adding versatility to your cooking. Both of these types of skillets are durable and can last a lifetime with proper care.

Sautéing is particularly well-suited for small, tender cuts of meat, seafood, and vegetables. For example, you can quickly sauté chicken breasts, shrimp, or thinly sliced beef for a fast and flavorful main dish. Vegetables like bell peppers, onions, and zucchini also take well to sautéing, developing a savory profile in just a few minutes.

Mastering the art of sautéing can open up a world of culinary possibilities for home cooks. Whether preparing a quick weeknight meal or adding a finishing touch to a more elaborate dish, sautéing is a versatile technique that delivers delicious results.

Simmering

Simmering is a gentle method that involves cooking a liquid at a temperature just below boiling, typically between 185°F and 205°F. This method allows food to cook slowly and evenly, developing deep flavors and tender textures without the risk of overcooking or breaking apart.

To simmer food properly, it's essential to maintain a consistent, low temperature. The liquid should have small, gentle bubbles that rise to the surface but do not break vigorously, as seen in boiling. Using a heavy-bottomed pot to distribute heat evenly and prevent scorching is essential. Adjusting the heat on the stove and occasionally stirring the pot will help maintain a steady simmer.

Simmering is particularly well-suited for dishes that benefit from long, slow cooking. This includes soups, stews, stocks, and braises. For example, simmering a beef stew makes the meat tender, and the flavors meld beautifully over time. Simmering helps extract all the flavors from the bones and vegetables when making homemade chicken stock, resulting in a rich, flavorful broth.

Smoking

Smoking is a cooking method that uses low heat and smoke to cook and flavor food simultaneously. This technique is ideal for meats, fish, and some vegetables, imparting a deep smoky flavor that other cooking methods can't replicate. The process involves exposing food to smoke from burning wood.

The history of smoking meat dates back thousands of years. Early humans discovered that smoking food added flavor and preserved it, allowing them to store food for extended periods. This was particularly useful before the advent of refrigeration. Over time, smoking techniques were refined, and today, it's a cherished tradition in many cultures, from American barbecue to Scandinavian smoked fish.

To smoke food properly, you need the right equipment and materials.

Types of smokers:

Offset Smokers:

This type of smoker features a firebox on the side of the smoking chamber. It's the best type of smoker as it allows the smoke to penetrate the meat without exposing it directly to the heat of the fire. This is my preferred type of smoker, and it's what the professionals use to produce some of the world's best barbecue.

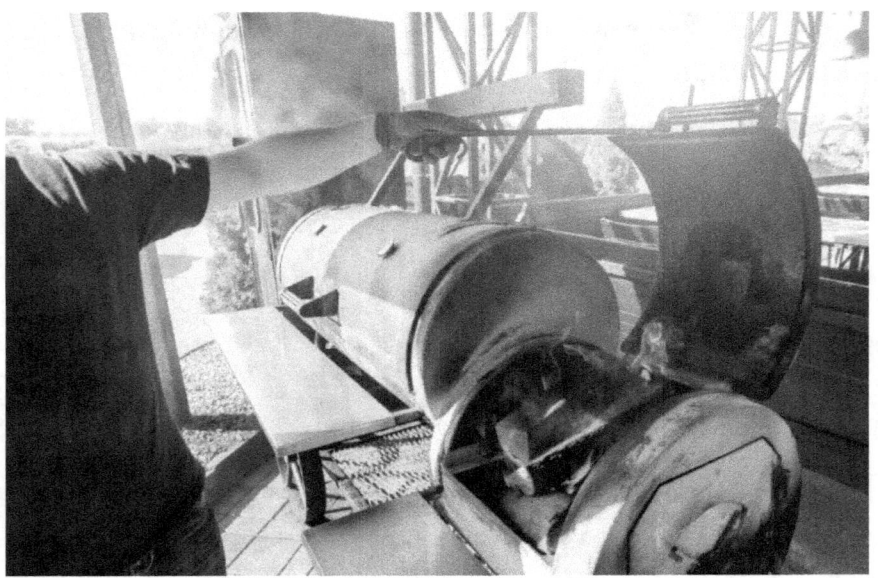

Smoking With a Gas Grill:

Smoking meat with a gas grill is possible, but it can be challenging. Placing a foil pouch with wood chips inside directly over a burner set on low heat and placing your meat on the opposite side of the grill with the burner off allows the smoke to penetrate the meat without overcooking it. Unless you have a large grill, it can quickly get overcrowded and won't leave room for much meat. You may have to replace your foil pouch several times depending on your smoke time and ensure the temperature stays low to find success with this method.

Electric Pellet Smokers:

These are easy to use and maintain consistent temperatures, making them ideal for beginners. They use an electric heating element and compressed wood pellets to produce the heat and smoke. They offer precise temperature control and are convenient for long smoking sessions. However, the pellets can be expensive and could contain undesirable filler materials.

When selecting wood for smoking, choosing the right type for the food you're cooking is essential. Hardwoods like hickory, oak, and mesquite provide bold flavors, while fruitwoods like apple, cherry, and maple offer milder, sweeter notes. Avoid using softwoods like pine or cedar, as they contain resins that can impart an unpleasant taste.

Smoking is particularly well-suited for larger cuts of meat that benefit from slow, low-heat cooking. This includes brisket, pork shoulder, ribs, and whole poultry. The long cooking time allows the smoke to penetrate deeply, creating layers of flavor. Fish, such as salmon and trout, also take well to smoking, developing a rich, smoky taste. Even vegetables like peppers, onions, and tomatoes can be enhanced with a touch of smoke.

For home cooks, smoking can seem intimidating at first, but with the right equipment and a bit of practice, it can become a rewarding and enjoyable method of cooking.

In summary, smoking is a time-honored cooking method that uses low heat and wood smoke to create deeply flavored, tender dishes. By choosing the right smoker, selecting appropriate woods, and maintaining steady temperatures, you can master the art of smoking and bring a rich, smoky taste to your culinary creations.

COOKING FOR CHANGE:

Carnivore, keto, low-carb, or no-carb, whatever your diet looks like, eating high protein and fat with minimal to no carbohydrates has helped me and countless others regain their health. Whether you need to lose body fat, build muscle, maintain your current metabolic state, or cure lifestyle diseases like obesity, type two diabetes, or high blood pressure, eating the foods made from the recipes contained within this cookbook, along with exercise, will make your health goal a reality.

You know how unhealthy food from restaurants, fast food establishments, and premade foods are. It's easy to succumb to temptation, but if you can find the courage to stick with the protein lifestyle for at least thirty days, you can overcome your cravings for food that do not serve your health.

The longer you adhere to this lifestyle, the more you will crave these foods, and when you're at a party and they are serving cake, you won't even think twice about passing on it.

Start today! If you're not experienced in the kitchen, start with one out of five meatball recipes that are the easiest to prepare and take the least amount of time to cook. If you start slow and build a list of a few recipes you like, you can make them staple meals and make them regularly. Once you have a handful, you can experiment with new recipes to add to your regular rotation.

Now that you're educated on some basic cooking skills and cooking methods, it's time to practice them. I hope you enjoy these recipes as much as I have over the years. Food is such an important part of our culture, and cooking food for yourself and your loved ones is one of the best ways to improve health and share your love. We celebrate with food, the smell of our favorite dishes can transport us through time and make us feel like we are back in that moment. Create new moments to remember with these dishes by sharing them with people you love.

"You must be committed to cooking eighty to ninety percent of your own foods to see positive results."

BEEF

Beef is the most affordable, available, and nutrient-dense food. It has all of the essential amino acids in the right proportions and is bioavailable. This means that the meat from a cow is the ideal food for us, and the more we eat, the healthier we will be. I am referring specifically to whole cuts of beef, ground beef, and organ meats. If you ate head to tail, you could thrive on beef alone.

I love the flavor of beef, especially from cows grazed on pasture and only fed natural supplemental feeds as needed. It is a very different flavor compared to beef from cows that were finished on corn and soy. The nutrient profile is also different; grass-finished cows have a balanced omega fatty acid profile and are generally healthier than their factory-farmed brethren. This is due to the natural way these cows are raised. If you can afford grass-finished and naturally-raised beef, go for that, but any beef is better than no beef.

I have included a wide range of beef recipes in this cookbook, from beef jerky to Texas-style smoked brisket.

Ground Beef Breakfast Bowl

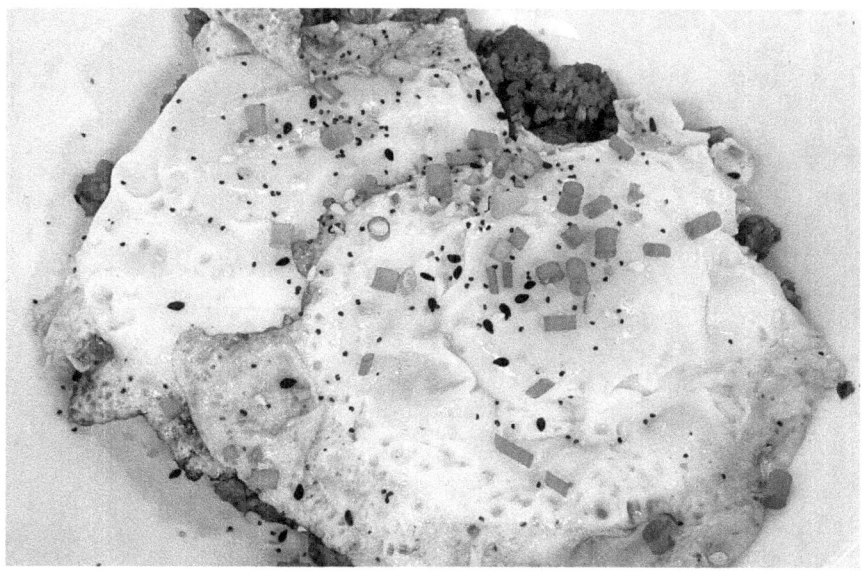

This hardy ground beef breakfast bowl recipe can be enjoyed any time of the day. It is an easy meal to prepare in advance by cooking a few pounds of ground beef and having it ready in the fridge. Then, when you are ready to eat, all you have to do is reheat the ground beef and cook the eggs. If you decide to cook the ground beef in advance, it will last up to one week in a sealed container in the fridge.

If you don't have a lid that fits your sauté pan, use aluminum foil, a plate, or a cutting board to cover it when cooking the eggs. I love this method because when you add water to the pan, the steam that is created will cook the top of the eggs; therefore, no flipping is required.

Add salt and any other seasoning while cooking the ground beef. Taco seasoning also works well in this dish. If you can't handle the heat, you can substitute the chili onion crunch with dehydrated onion; you'll still get a bit of a crunch without the spice.

Difficulty Level: 2 out of 5 Meatballs

Prep Time: 5 Minutes

Cook Time: 15 Minutes

Servings: 2

Nutritional Facts: (Per Serving)
Calories 957
Protein 52g
Fat 74g
Total Carbohydrates 16g

1 pound ground beef

4 eggs

1 tablespoon of butter

1 bunch of green onions, washed and sliced thin

1 tablespoon of everything bagel seasoning

1 tablespoon of chili onion crunch

1 teaspoon of salt

Add the ground beef to a large sauté pan and season with salt. Cook the ground beef over high heat until browned, then divide it into two medium-sized serving bowls.

Add the butter to the sauté pan over medium heat. Immediately after the butter melts, carefully crack the eggs into the pan and leave them to cook for 1 minute.

Then, add a splash of water to the pan surface, cover, and cook for another 2 minutes for medium-soft yolks.

Remove the eggs from the pan and place two eggs in each bowl on top of the ground beef.

Top with green onion, everything bagel seasoning, and chili onion crunch and enjoy.

Braised Beef Short Ribs with Red Wine Reduction

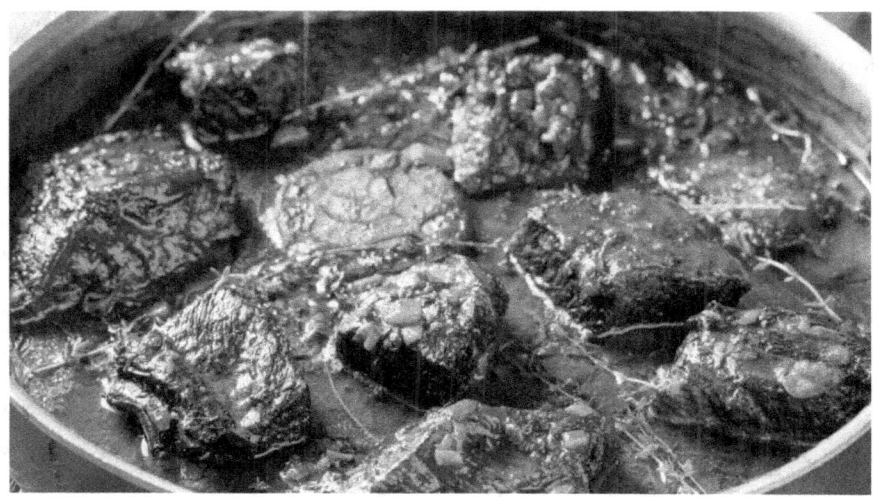

My braised beef short ribs with a red wine reduction is by far the most involved recipe in this cookbook, but all the effort will pay off. You will have a flavor experience like you have never had before with a home-cooked meal. Preparing the port wine reduction and aromatics in advance can make preparing this recipe easier.

Use English-cut short ribs for this recipe. English-cut short ribs are cut such that one rib bone runs along the length of each portion, whereas flanken-cut ribs are sliced across the ribs so that each piece has a cross-section of several rib bones.

Try to find English-cut short ribs that are about four inches in length and are well-marbled with a nice meaty portion on each rib.

This recipe calls for an instant pot, but it can be made in a pot with a lid. However, it will take a bit longer to braise the short ribs versus pressure cooking them.

Grilling the short ribs adds flavor to this dish. While it can also be done on a cast iron skillet, I find it faster and easier to clean up when using a grill.

Reducing the port wine to a syrup is simple. However, reducing the entire bottle to half a cup takes time. The more surface area you provide for this, the less time it will take to evaporate the water out of the wine.

When the ribs are removed from the pot, they will be very tender, and the bones may slip out; try to hold them together so they do not fall apart as you transfer them. You can also substitute the short ribs for a chuck roast if you so desire. Nevertheless, I would recommend a bone-in roast, as this will also add more flavor to the final dish.

You can enjoy this recipe as a stand-alone dish or with a side of mashed potatoes, or if your eating low- carb try it with a side of bacon twists found on page 149.

Difficulty Level: 5 out of 5 Meatballs

Prep Time: 2 Hours

Cook Time: 1 Hour

Servings: 5

Nutritional Facts:
(Per Serving)

Calories 993

Protein 68g

Fat 35g

Total Carbohydrates 29g

5 pounds of beef short ribs

2 celery ribs, washed and roughly chopped

2 large carrots, washed and roughly chopped

1 large yellow onion, washed and roughly chopped

1 bulb of garlic, washed and peeled

2 tablespoons of tomato paste

1 (750ml) bottle of dry red wine

1 quart of beef stock

4 sprigs of fresh thyme

2 bay leaves

1 (750ml) bottle of ruby port wine

1 tablespoon of Worcestershire sauce

1 tablespoon of coconut aminos

1 Shallot

Salt and fresh ground black pepper to taste

2 tablespoons of beef tallow or clarified butter

Allow the short ribs to come to room temperature. Preheat the grill to high. Season the short ribs with salt and pepper and grill for 3 minutes cn each side. Remove from heat and set aside.

Add 2 tablespoons of tallow or clarified butter to the instant pot and set to sauté mode on high. Once the pot is hot, add the celery and carrots. Cook for 5 minutes, stirring every few minutes.

Add the onion and shallots to the pot, sprinkle with a pinch of salt, and continue cooking for another 3 minutes, stirring every few minutes. Then, stir in the garlic and continue cooking for another minute.

Stir in the tomato paste and cook for 1 minute longer; lower heat at any point if the contents of the pot threaten to burn. Pour in the dry red wine and scrape up any browned bits from the bottom and sides of the pot. Let the mixture come to a simmer, then add the beef stock, coconut aminos, Worcestershire sauce, and a pinch of salt and pepper. Stir to mix.

Add the short ribs, thyme, and bay leaves to the pot. Pressure cook on high for 45 minutes, with a 15-minute natural pressure release.

Meanwhile, in a large saucepan, bring the port wine to a very gentle simmer, regulating heat to maintain. Cook, uncovered, to reduce until syrupy, about 1 hour; should yield about 1/2 cup in volume and set aside.

Once the ribs are done, carefully remove them and place them on a clean platter, tenting with foil. Strain the braising liquid through a fine-mesh strainer over a large bowl, pressing on the solids to extract as much liquid as possible.

Rinse out the pot and return the strained braising liquid to it. Return to heat and bring to a gentle simmer until the braising liquid is reduced to 2 cups. This should take about 1 hour; skim any foam that accumulates on the surface as needed.

Add the port wine reduction to the braising liquid. The sauce should be thick enough to coat the back of a spoon.

Season the sauce with salt and pepper to taste. Return the short ribs to the pot, spoon the sauce over and around to glaze and rewarm them, and indulge in the complex flavors and tenderness!

Teriyaki Beef

This version of teriyaki beef is soy-free and does not use any added sugar. Instead, it calls for coconut aminos made from the fermented sap of the coconut palm.

I have included a roasted broccoli recipe following this one, so you can make beef and broccoli or use it as a side with another recipe. If you follow a less strict carnivore diet, the teriyaki beef recipe will work for you, and if you are eating keto, you can combine these recipes to make a fantastic meal.

The longer you marinate the beef, the more flavorful and tender it will be, but an hour will do if you're short on time. If you have a vacuum sealer, you can vacuum seal the beef in the marinade to impart even more flavor to the meat.

The teriyaki beef will last in the fridge for up to a week and, if frozen, for three months.

Try adding dried pepper flakes or garlic chili sauce for some added heat.

I use beef bottom round steak that is a quarter-inch thick. I cut it into one-inch-wide strips. You can use many other cuts of beef, such as flank or skirt steak.

To reduce preparation time, consider using premade frozen garlic and ginger cubes.

This teriyaki beef and broccoli is an excellent meal alone, but it can also be served with sautéed onions and bell peppers for a more stir-fry-style dish.

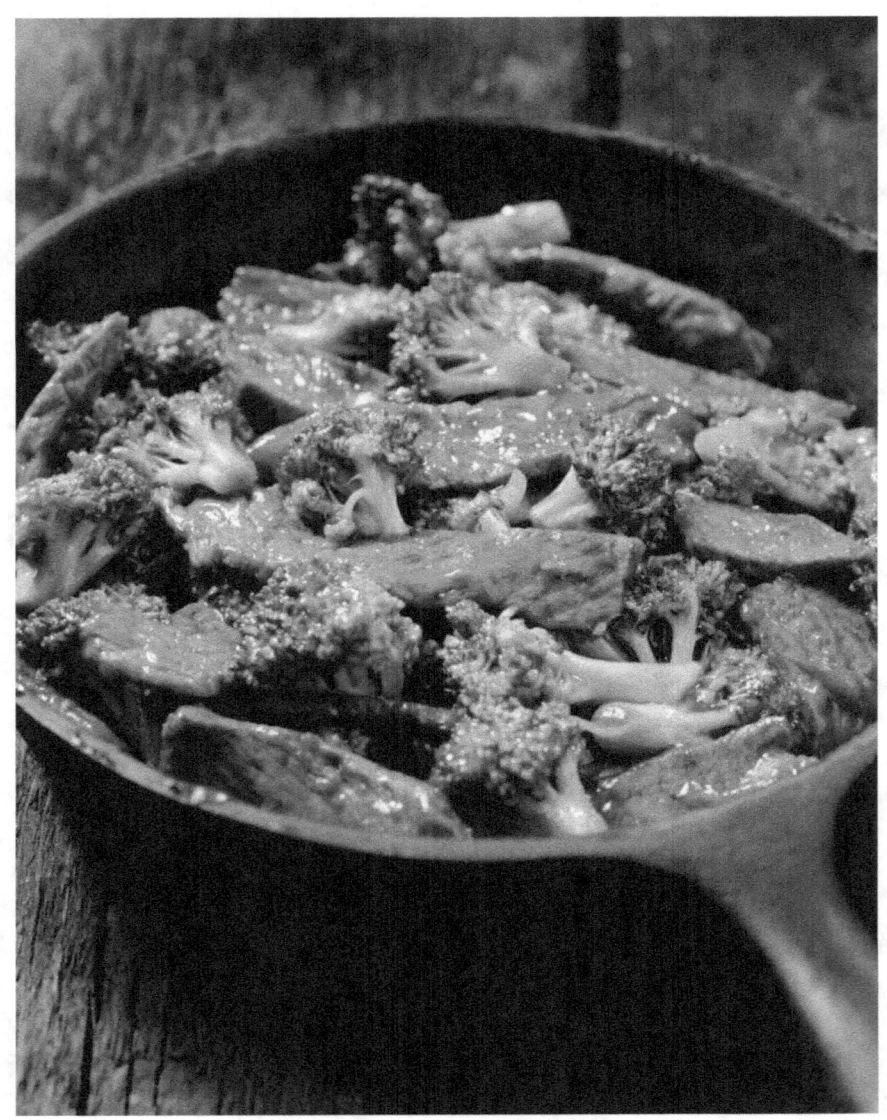

Difficulty Level: 3 out of 5 Meatballs

Prep Time: 5 Minutes

Cook Time: 10 Minutes

Servings: 4

Nutritional Facts:
(Per Serving)

Calories 617

Protein 76g

Fat 28g

Total Carbohydrates

2 tablespoons of rice vinegar

2-3 pounds of beef bottom round steak, ¼ inch thick, cut into 1-inch wide strips

1/2 cup of coconut aminos

2 cloves of garlic, minced

1 inch of ginger root, grated

1 tablespoon of Worcestershire sauce

2 tablespoons of coconut oil

1 tablespoon of sesame oil

1 tablespoon of toasted sesame seeds

1 teaspoon of salt

2 teaspoons of pepper

Place the beef in a large container. Add 1 tablespoon of rice vinegar and 1/4 cup of coconut aminos and mix to coat the beef. Refrigerate for at least one hour, or overnight for best results.

Prepare the sauce in a small bowl by combining the remaining rice vinegar, coconut aminos, and the sesame oil, ginger, garlic, and Worcestershire sauce. Stir to mix, and set aside.

Remove beef from marinade and let it come to room temperature.

Place a large skillet over high heat, and add the coconut oil. Once the pan is hot, add the beef and stir every few minutes until it is fully cooked and slightly charred.

To serve, toss a portion of the beef in the sauce and enjoy!

Roasted Broccoli

Difficulty Level: 1 out of 5 Meatballs

Prep Time: 5 Minutes

Cook Time: 20 Minutes

Servings: 4

Nutritional Facts:
(Per Serving)
Calories 117
Protein 4g
Fat 8g
Total Carbohydrates 10g

1 head of broccoli, cut into bite-size pieces

2 tablespoons of clarified butter, melted

½ teaspoon of salt

¼ teaspoon of pepper

Preheat your oven to 425°F.

Toss the broccoli florets and clarified butter in a large bowl.

Spread the broccoli on a baking sheet and sprinkle with the salt and pepper.

Bake for 15-20 or until the edges start to brown.

Steak Three-Ways:
Grill, Air fry, or Pan-Fry Your Way to Perfection

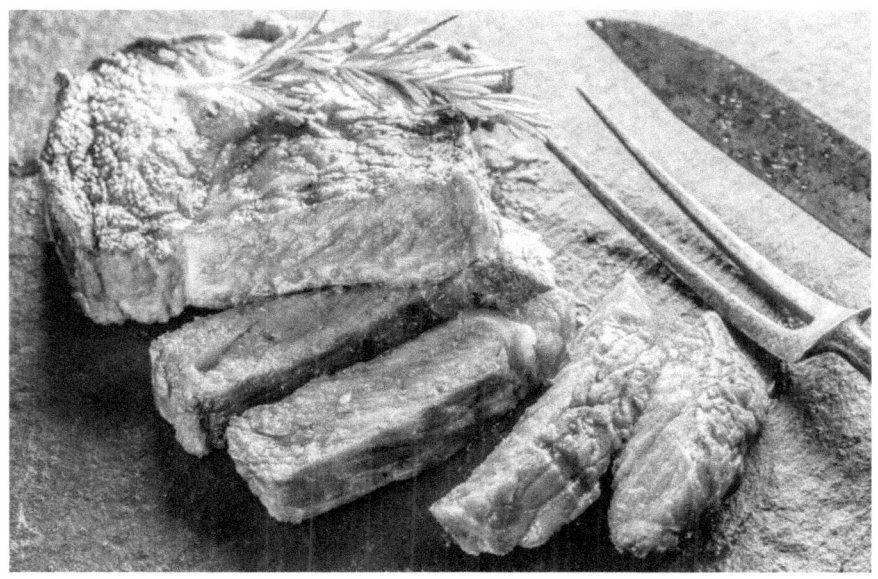

Steak is one of my favorite foods. It's easy to make, tastes fantastic, and can be made at home for a fraction of the price of a fancy steak house. Beef is incredibly nutritious, and those nutrients are in the proper proportions and bioavailable so our bodies can utilize them fully. It is truly a superfood.

Humans have been cooking meat for as long as we have had fire, so we've been at it a while, but not much has changed. A good steak only requires a little salt and a few minutes over a fire to create a fantastic meal.

Let your steak come to room temperature by removing it from the fridge for at least one hour before cooking. This will allow your steak to cook more evenly. If the steak is cold when you cook it, you may overcook the outer surface and still have it raw in the middle.

You will need a meat thermometer to check the doneness of your steak. There are several types available. The most common are the standard digital probe, cord or cordless probe, or the classic old-school bi-metallic thermometer. It doesn't matter which kind you use as long as it is accurate. You can always cut the steak open to check for doneness in a pinch, but that only works once, will release the juices from the meat, and can contribute to dryness.

This recipe calls for a ten-ounce New York strip steak that is one inch thick. This is because when you use the air fryer method, you need a thicker steak to prevent it from overcooking. However, you can use any thickness or cut of steak you like if you choose the grill or pan fry method. The thicker it is, the longer you must cook it. Some good options are ribeye, porterhouse, or skirt steak.

Cooking time by thickness:

Thin (1/2 inch or smaller): 1 minute or less per side

Medium: (1/2 inch to 1 inch): 2 minutes per side

Thick (1 inch or more): 3 minutes or more per side

Remember that these are average cooking times, and a meat thermometer should be used in conjunction with the included temperature chart to determine when a steak is ready. Keeping your cooking surface nice and hot will help add beautiful sear marks to your steak. After you have achieved the sear, you only need to worry about the internal temperature.

Steak is best eaten fresh but can be stored in your fridge for about a week. If you make your steak beforehand, undercook it so it will not overcook when you reheat it.

A good steak requires nothing more than salt and maybe some pepper, but you have a few options if you want to add more flavor. You can marinate thinner cuts to help tenderize them and add flavor. You could also include additional seasoning like onion or garlic powder. When pan-frying your steak, add garlic and fresh herbs like rosemary or thyme during cooking.

I have included a recipe for my blue cheese sauce following this recipe. It is incredible with any steak; don't skip it, or you will regret it.

Cooking steak is simple. Get your cooking surface hot to get a good sear on the outside, then monitor the internal temperature with a meat thermometer. Pull it from the heat as soon as it reaches the "remove from heat temperature" and let it rest for five minutes. That's it!

Steak is excellent all on its own, but some grilled vegetables will pair well with it if you want to add some variety. A compound butter would also enhance the flavor of your steak and can be prepared quickly by mixing softened butter with herbs and spices. Or you can do what I do when I'm feeling fancy and dip each bit of steak in some melted browned butter!

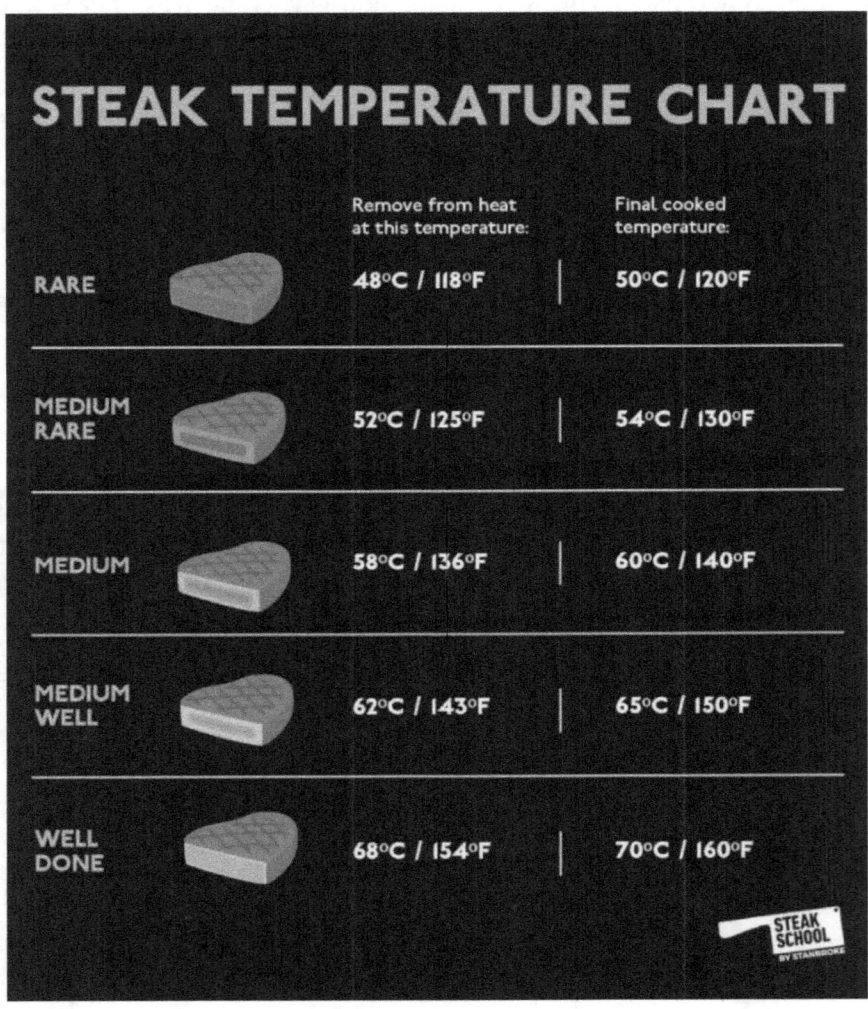

Difficulty Level: 2 out of 5 Meatballs

Prep Time: 5 Minutes

Cook Time: 6-18 Minutes

Servings: 1

Nutritional Facts:
(Per Serving)

Calories 735

Protein 58g

Fat 53g

Total Carbohydrates

1 ten-ounce New York strip steak, one inch thick

1 tablespoon of course sea salt

1 tablespoon of butter, room temperature

Remove your steak from the fridge for at least one hour before cooking to let it come to room temperature.

Pat the steak dry with paper towels and liberally sprinkle with salt on both sides.

Grill Method

Preheat the grill to high. Once hot, clean the grill.

Grill steak for about three minutes on each side.

Air Fry Method

Preheat the air fryer to 400°F.

Defrosted

Air fry at 400°F for 6 minutes on each side.

Frozen

Air fry at 400°F for 9 minutes on each side.

Pan-Fry Method

Clarify the butter. Directions for this can be found on page 107.

Place a large-sized skillet over high heat and add the clarified butter.

Once the skillet is hot but not smoking, add the steak.

Cook the steak for 3 minutes on each side.

Checking for Doneness

To check the temperature, insert a meat thermometer into the thickest part of the steak (see temperature guide).

When cooked to your desired temperature, remove from heat and let rest for 5 minutes.

Serve on a warm plate, and place the butter or a compound butter on top of the steak or eat with the blue cheese sauce and enjoy!

Blue Cheese Sauce

You will never want to eat another steak without this blue cheese sauce! It's quick to whip up and has nine grams of protein per serving.

The base of this recipe is cottage cheese. I wanted a sauce with no ultra-processed oils or high fructose corn syrup, as most store bought sauces have. So as I do, I made my own.

You will need a blender or food processor to process the cottage cheese into a liquid properly, but a blender or food processor of any size will work. The key to this recipe is processing the mixture until it is velvety smooth.

This recipe can be made beforehand but will only last three to five days in the fridge.

Difficulty Level: 1 out of 5 Meatballs

Prep Time: 5 Minutes

Cook Time: None

Servings: 4

Nutritional Facts: (Per Serving)
Calories 114
Protein 9g
Fat 7g
Total Carbohydrates

One cup of cottage cheese

6 tablespoons of water

2.5 ounces of blue cheese

Place ingredients into a blender and blend on high for 1 minute.

Use a rubber spatula to scrape down the sides of the blender pitcher.

Blend until smooth.

Serve with steak or use as a dip.

Low-Carb Meatloaf

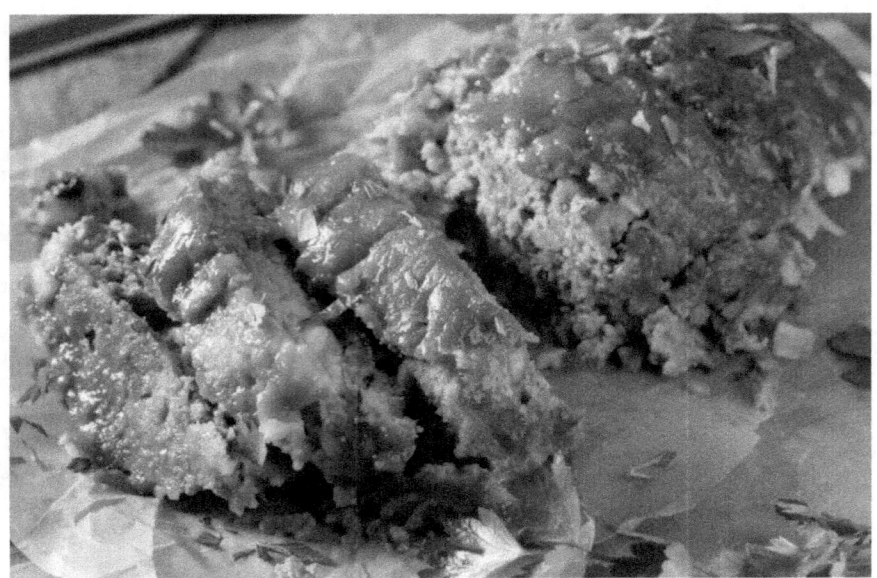

This low-carb meatloaf recipe is a take on the classic meatloaf, but it features pork panko instead of bread crumbs and includes a recipe for homemade ketchup with no added sugars, so you can enjoy it whether you're eating keto or not.

A loaf pan is required to make this recipe. You could use another type of pan, but you will want to use a narrow one, or you risk drying out your meatloaf.

When you add the meat mixture to the loaf pan, shape the meatloaf with your hands. First, level the mixture in the pan and then push down on all of the edges to create a raised center similar to a loaf of bread.

If you have more meat mixture than will fit in your pan or want to mix it up, make mini meatloaf muffins in a muffin pan or silicone muffin liners. Add the ketchup glaze and bake them for 18-20 minutes.

You could substitute the ketchup glaze for a layer of your cheese of choice and top with green onions, or add bacon crumbles for added flavor.

Your meatloaf is done when the ketchup glaze starts to brown slightly. Caramelizing the sugars adds a fantastic depth of flavor and improves the plate's presentation.

You can store your meatloaf in an airtight container in the fridge for up to one week or freeze it for up to three months.

You can also create an Asian-inspired meatloaf by replacing the Italian seasoning with fresh grated ginger and adding coconut aminos. Then, substitute the ketchup glaze with your favorite Korean barbeque sauce.

Difficulty Level: 3 out of 5 Meatballs

Prep Time: 10 Minutes

Cook Time: 1 Hour

Servings: 6

Nutritional Facts:
(Per Serving)

Calories 653

Protein 43g

Fat 48g

Total Carbohydrates

3 pounds of 80/20 ground beef

4 eggs

1/4 cup of pork panko

1 tablespoon of Italian seasoning

2 tablespoons of parsley, washed and chopped

1/2 medium onion, washed and grated

4 cloves of garlic, minced

1 tablespoon of Worcestershire sauce

2 tablespoons of salt

1/2 teaspoon of black pepper

Preheat the oven to 375°F. Line a 9x5-inch loaf pan with parchment paper and set aside.

Combine all the ingredients in a large mixing bowl and mix well. Add the meatloaf mixture to the loaf pan and shape it into a loaf.

Bake for 40 minutes. While the meatloaf is baking, prepare the ketchup glaze.

After 40 minutes, remove the meatloaf, spread the ketchup glaze on top, and bake for 15-20 minutes.

Remove the meatloaf from the oven, let it rest for 10 minutes, and garnish with fresh parsley. Slice and enjoy!

Homemade Ketchup

Most commercially available ketchup is made with high fructose corn syrup, so I have included this no-sugar-added homemade ketchup recipe.

To check the ketchup's flavor, once reduced, remove a spoonful from the saucepan and let it cool on the counter. You'll want to taste it after it has cooled for an accurate adjustment. Taste and adjust if desired, adding salt to taste, more vinegar for tang, more maple syrup for sweetness, or more onion powder for additional savory notes.

Your homemade ketchup will store in the fridge for up to 2 weeks or in the freezer for up to 2 months. If freezing, consider using an ice cube tray. This way, it will defrost faster, and you can defrost only as much as you need at a time.

This ketchup goes well with French fries fried in tallow or as tomato sauce on pizza. However, I would reduce the amount of maple syrup for this application.

A half batch of this ketchup recipe is enough for one meatloaf.

Difficulty Level: 2 out of 5 Meatballs

Prep Time: 5 Minutes

Cook Time: 1 Hour

Servings: 12

Nutritional Facts:
(Per Serving)

Calories 37

Protein 0.5g

Fat 0g

Total Carbohydrates

---

12 ounces of tomato purée

1/3 cup of maple syrup

1/4 cup of white vinegar

2 tablespoons of apple cider vinegar

1/2 teaspoon of onion powder

1 teaspoon of garlic powder

1 teaspoon of sea salt

Place all ingredients in a medium saucepan, stir until well combined, turn the heat on medium. Stir gently until everything comes to a light simmer, then reduce heat to low.

Let simmer for 30-45 minutes or until slightly reduced and darkened in color, stirring every 5 minutes to prevent sticking.

Remove from heat and let cool for 5 minutes before serving.

Ground Beef Kefta Kebabs

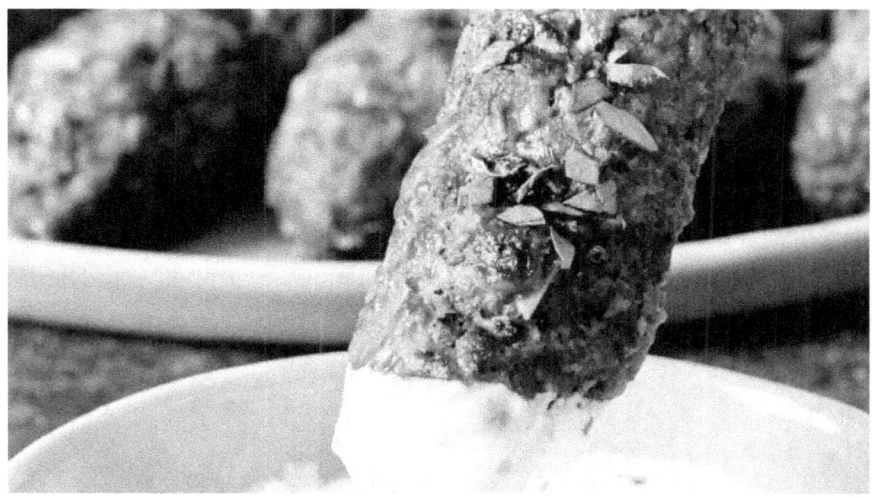

I can't get enough of these ground beef kefta kebabs. I enjoy the unique Moroccan flavor this dish brings to the table, and the tzatziki sauce adds a fantastic layer of flavor that pairs perfectly.

A blender or food processor makes crafting the recipe a breeze, but if you don't have either, you could prepare everything by hand or with a box grater. Just make sure to chop everything very finely so there are no big chunks of anything.

When forming the kebabs, wetting your hands so the meat mixture does not stick to them can be helpful. I find it easiest to form a ball and then roll it back and forth between my hands to get that classic kebab shape. Then all you have to do is thread it on the skewer and make sure the tip is not poking out the end of the kebab.

If using wooden skewers, soak them in water for at least 15 minutes before threading the meat onto them so they do not burn as much when grilling.

If you do not have a grill, these kebobs can be cooked in a sauté pan over the stove or on a baking sheet in the oven. Add olive oil to prevent your kebobs from sticking and ditch the skewers.

The grilled kebabs can be stored in the fridge for about one week or frozen for up to three months.

By placing the meat mixture in the fridge before you make the kebabs, you allow it to firm up. This will help them retain their shape during the cooking process. It also allows the flavors to combine, which can make for a more flavorful dining experience.

These kebabs are best served with basmati rice, pita bread, and hummus. Some sliced vegetables like cucumber, tomato, and onion also pair well. If you are eating a low-carb diet, you can substitute the basmati rice with cauliflower rice or just eat the kebobs with the tzatziki sauce.

Difficulty Level: 4 out of 5 Meatballs

Prep Time: 30 Minutes

Cook Time: 10 Minutes

Servings: 2

Nutritional Facts:
(Per Serving)

Calories 627

Protein 40g

Fat 46g

Total Carbohydrates 10g

1 pound of ground beef or lamb

1 medium onion, grated

3 cloves garlic, peeled and finely chopped

2 teaspoons of paprika

1 teaspoon of ground cumin

2 teaspoons of ground coriander

1 teaspoon of salt

1/4 teaspoon of pepper

1/8 teaspoon of cayenne pepper

1/4 cup of fresh parsley, washed and chopped

1/4 cup of fresh cilantro, washed and chopped

1/2 teaspoon of cinnamon

1 tablespoon of fresh mint, washed and chopped

Soak the wooden skewers in water until needed.

Combine all the ingredients in a large bowl and mix by hand until well combined. Refrigerate the mixture for at least.

Preheat your grill. Divide the mixture into 6 portions and mold each into a tubular shape like a sausage. Thread each onto a skewer.

Just before you grill the kebabs, brush the grill lightly with olive oil to prevent sticking. Grill the kebabs for about 5 minutes on each side.

Let cool for 5 minutes, serve with tzatziki sauce, and enjoy!

Tzatziki Sauce

This tzatziki sauce is so refreshing and delicious that you'll want to put it on more than just your kefta kebobs. This recipe is simple and easy to prepare. If you don't like mint, try substituting it for dill.

Difficulty Level: 1 out of 5 Meatballs

Prep Time: 5 Minutes

Cook Time: None

Servings: 2

Nutritional Facts:
(Per Serving)

Calories 74

Protein 10g

Fat .50g

Total Carbohydrates

1 cup of plain Greek yogurt

2 Persian cucumbers, washed

2 cloves of garlic, peeled

1 teaspoon of lemon juice

1 teaspoon of fresh mint (1/4 teaspoon dried)

1/8 teaspoon of salt

Grate the cucumbers with a box grater. Using a strainer, press as much moisture out of the grated cucumber as possible.

Place all of the ingredients into a food processor or blender and blend until all of the ingredients are combined and form a smooth uniform consistency.

Refrigerate the mixture for a minimum of one hour to allow it to thicken before serving.

Blue Cheese and Bacon Beast Burgers

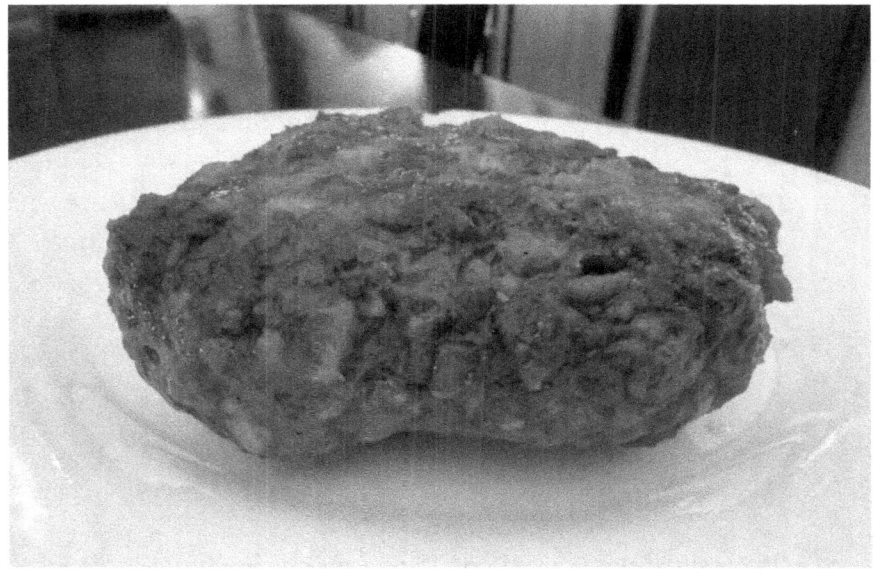

This recipe is a take on the classic hamburger. It's high in fat and protein, and I have included an additional recipe for carnivore buns that pairs very nicely with this recipe.

You can use your hands to form the patties, a burger press, or a plate to press your burger to create a uniform patty. If you do this, place a piece of parchment paper on top and bottom to avoid the meat sticking. If your patties become deformed, you can always reshape them by hand.

You usually let the meat come to room temperature before cooking, but this is not the case for hamburgers. As the temperature of the ground beef rises, the fat will become less solid, making working with it more difficult. So when you make your hamburgers, leave the ground beef in the fridge until just before you make the patties. For this very reason, you should refrigerate the patties before grilling them.

This recipe pairs well with my Homemade Ketchup, found on page 51.

Difficulty Level: 3 out of 5 Meatballs

Prep Time: 5 Minutes

Cook Time: 10 Minutes

Servings: 2

Nutritional Facts: (Per Serving)
Calories 1149
Protein 59g
Fat 98g
Total Carbohydrates

1 pound of ground beef

½ pound of bacon, crumbled and extra crispy

2.5 ounces of blue cheese crumbles

1 teaspoon salt

Place all of the ingredients in a large mixing bowl. Mix by hand until all ingredients are well incorporated.

Divide the meat mixture into 4 parts and then form each into about 1-inch thick patties.

Refrigerate the patties for at least 20 minutes before grilling to let them firm up.

Grill the patties on a barbecue grill or in a skillet over high heat for about 5 minutes on each side or until they reach an internal temperature of 160 ° Fahrenheit.

Let your burgers cool for 5 minutes, serve, and enjoy!

Carnivore Buns

These carnivore buns have under one gram of carbohydrates, are savory, and hold up well, making them perfect for eating with hamburgers.

This recipe was adapted from a carnivore tortilla recipe that I found to be too thick to use as tortillas. I modified the recipe to make them a fantastic substitute for sandwich bread or hamburger buns.

If you're unfamiliar with pork panko, it's made from crushed pork rinds. I have included instructions on making this in my turkey nugget recipe, which can be found on page 156.

Greasing the back of a spoon to spread/ shape your buns will help keep the batter from sticking to it. Use butter, tallow, or bacon drippings for this. Use the back of your greased spoon to spread the batter in the skillet in a circular motion, and pull the spoon away to the side rather than straight up to help avoid it from sticking. The butter in the batter will help to keep your buns from sticking to the skillet.

The batter will be thick. You will need to use two spoons to get it into the skillet. These buns can be stored in your fridge for up to one week.

Difficulty Level: 2 out of 5 Meatballs

Prep Time: 5 Minutes

Cook Time: 4-8 Minutes

Servings: 1

Nutritional Facts:
(Per Serving)
Calories 557
Protein 37g
Fat 44g
Total Carbohydrates 0g

1/2 cup pork panko

2 eggs

2 tablespoons of butter, melted

Add half of the bun batter to a skillet and spread it out with the back of a greased spoon.

Cook for one to two minutes on each side and remove from heat.

Repeat this process with the second half of the batter.

Let your buns cool for 3 minutes, and enjoy.

Beef Jerky

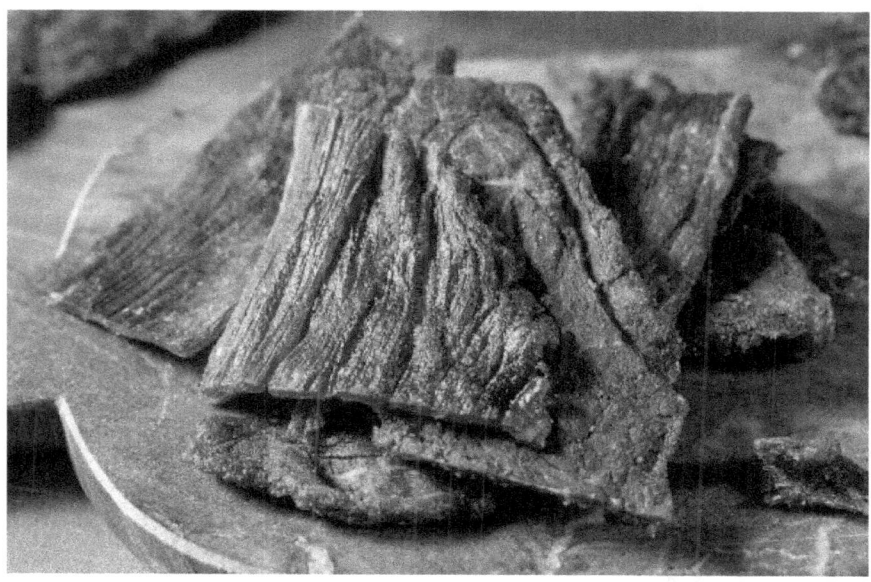

The ultimate portable protein beef jerky was a staple of pioneers and adventurers throughout time and is still enjoyed worldwide by many cultures. Its lightweight and highly nutritious nature makes it perfect for fueling up on the go. You can snack on this delicious food on the trail, while traveling, or anytime you need to satiate your hunger.

The tradition of preserving meat goes back thousands of years. Preserving meat in this fashion was widespread before refrigeration, as meat would spoil in only a few days at room temperature. However, if you could dry your meat by smoking or placing it near a fire, it could be made to last much longer.

You don't need any special equipment to make beef jerky, but there are some advantages to using a dehydrator versus an oven. For one, dehydrators offer a stable temperature and are less likely to over or under-dry the end product. Additionally, dehydrators have a built-in fan to help remove additional moisture. You can also use a convection oven to get the same effect.

Removing as much moisture as possible is essential to avoid spoilage. Another key to preserving meats is removing as much fat as possible, as fat contains a lot of water, which can contribute to mold.

You will want to use lean cuts of beef, like top or bottom round or an eye of round roast. You can buy thin-cut steaks that are 1/8 to 1/4 inches thick or slice a roast yourself. If you cut your own, one tip is to put the roast in the freezer for an hour before you slice it. Doing this firms up the meat, making it easier to slice it thin. Cut the roast against the grain when slicing to avoid chewy beef jerky.

Well-dried beef jerky can last up to a year or longer at room temperature, but it is not as enjoyable as medium-dried jerky, which is what this recipe aims to achieve. You can dry it longer if you want it to last longer or store it in the fridge.

Most jerky on grocery store shelves and in gas stations are loaded with sugar and other preservatives, artificial flavors, and other harmful chemicals. It could be a better option than ultra-processed protein bars, but it's better for your gut not to consume these things when you can.

Even most homemade beef jerky recipes use ingredients that are not health-promoting, like sugar and artificial smoke flavoring. This recipe has none of that garbage and tastes better, too.

This is a basic recipe to introduce you to the practice of preserving meat, but you can mix it up and customize it to your particular tastes. Add some red pepper flakes and fresh ground black pepper if you like spicy food. I also recommend total seasoning.

Many recipes call to marinate your beef before dehydration, and soy sauce is primarily used as a base. I try to avoid soy as much as possible due to its estrogenic properties, and I recommend you do the same; nevertheless, if you want to try marinating your beef to get another layer of flavor, try using coconut aminos, apple cider vinegar, Worcestershire sauce, garlic powder, onion powder, and pepper. Coconut aminos do contain sugar, but it's in a more natural state than cane sugar.

Try using balsamic vinaigrette, pineapple juice, and, you guessed it, coconut aminos for a unique flavor experience. Marinate your beef for an hour or even overnight in the fridge for maximum flavor. Beef jerky tends to be dryer in Mexico, and it's a popular practice to add lemon juice and tajin to this style of beef jerky to moisten it and add some spice.

There is more than just beef jerky. Turkey, chicken, and even pork jerky are options, but using these meats presents a more significant challenge due to their different fat ratios.

The key to making jerky that lasts is getting all the moisture out. One tip is to use a fan to completely dry and cool your jerky before you store it.

Beef jerky is a convenient snack that you can take on the go and enjoy anytime you need some vital protein.

Difficulty Level: 1 out of 5 Meatballs

Prep Time: 5 Minutes

Cook Time: 3-4 Hours

Servings: 6

Nutritional Facts:
(Per Serving)
Calories 317
Protein 50g
Fat 11g
Total Carbohydrates

3 pounds of lean beef, thinly sliced (1/8 and 1/4 inch thick)

1 tablespoon of fine salt

Preheat your oven to 175°F.

Dry the beef with a paper towel. Sprinkle salt on both sides of the beef slices and place them on a baking sheet or baking rack.

Bake at 175°F for 3-4 hours, flipping the slices every hour to ensure even drying.

Check your beef at 3 hours to determine if it is done. Do this by taking a piece out of the oven and letting it cool for a few minutes. It should be dry to the touch, leather-like in appearance, and chewy but still somewhat tender.

If it's not done, put it back in the oven and check it every 30 minutes.

Once your beef jerky is dehydrated, dry off any grease that may have accumulated on the meat and let it cool on your countertop for at least an hour before storing it in an airtight container.

Stovetop Popcorn

Growing up, my mom often took my sisters and me to the movie theater. We loved it, but honestly, the biggest draw was the coveted movie theater popcorn. Popcorn was also a staple snack at home during my childhood, whether it was microwaved or the less popular air-popped or "healthy" version.

Movie theater, microwave, and prepackaged popcorn contain unfavorable oils and artificial flavors that are not good for you, so if you want to enjoy this high-carb snack, you need to make it yourself to mitigate the unhealthy aspects.

I have paired this popcorn recipe with my beef jerky recipe to help you meet your protein requirements. Since popcorn is very low in protein, eating these items together makes you more likely to hit your protein goal for the day. All you have to do is eat the beef jerky first, and then you can enjoy the popcorn guilt-free.

There are tons of gadgets available to make popcorn, from air poppers to pressure poppers used by street vendors in China. These gadgets can be fun to use but also take up space on your countertop or in your cabinet. You can make it in a metal bowl and use aluminum foil with holes punched in it to allow the steam to vent. I like to use a cast iron Dutch oven with a lid, but any pot with a lid will do.

Venting the steam will help avoid soggy popcorn, so crack the lid a little but not too much or you will have popped corn all over the place.

Popcorn is best enjoyed hot and fresh, but it can also be made in advance and stored in an airtight container to prevent it from going stale.

When it comes to flavoring your popped corn, you have many options, from the traditional salt and butter to Asian-inspired popcorn using furikake sushi seasoning. An easy way to add butter is to throw a tablespoon of butter in the pan just as the kernels start to pop. The butter will melt and be incorporated into the popcorn as it pops.

Other topping ideas include:

Cheese Powder

Chili Lime Seasoning

Everything Bagel Seasoning

Lowry's Seasoning Salt

Nutritional Yeast

Ranch Dip Powder

The finer, the better when it comes to toppings. Fine salt will adhere to the popcorn much better than course salts; this is the same for any topping.

You also have options for the type of cooking fat you use. The fat you choose will impart additional flavor. I like coconut oil due to its health-promoting properties and unique flavor. However, you could also try tallow, sesame seed oil, or even bacon grease. Any high-heat oil or fat will work.

The sky is the limit when it comes to choosing how to flavor your popcorn. Once you have the standard recipe down, feel free to experiment with different combinations of toppings and fats to see what you like best.

Difficulty Level: 1 out of 5 Meatballs

Prep Time: 5 Minutes

Cook Time: 3-4 Minutes

Servings: 2

Nutritional Facts:
(Per Serving)

Calories 317

Protein 50g

Fat 11g

Total Carbohydrates

1 tablespoons coconut oil

1/3 cup organic popcorn kernels

Fine salt to taste

Place a medium size pot over high heat and add the coconut oil and popcorn kernels.

Once the oil has melted, swirl the pot a few times to coat the kernels with oil. Cover the pan with a lid, leaving a small opening to allow the steam to vent. The kernels will start popping in a minute or two.

Once the popping slows to about 8 seconds between pops, immediately dump the popcorn into a big bowl, sprinkle with salt.

Let it cool for one minute, and enjoy.

Basil and Ricotta Meatball Casserole

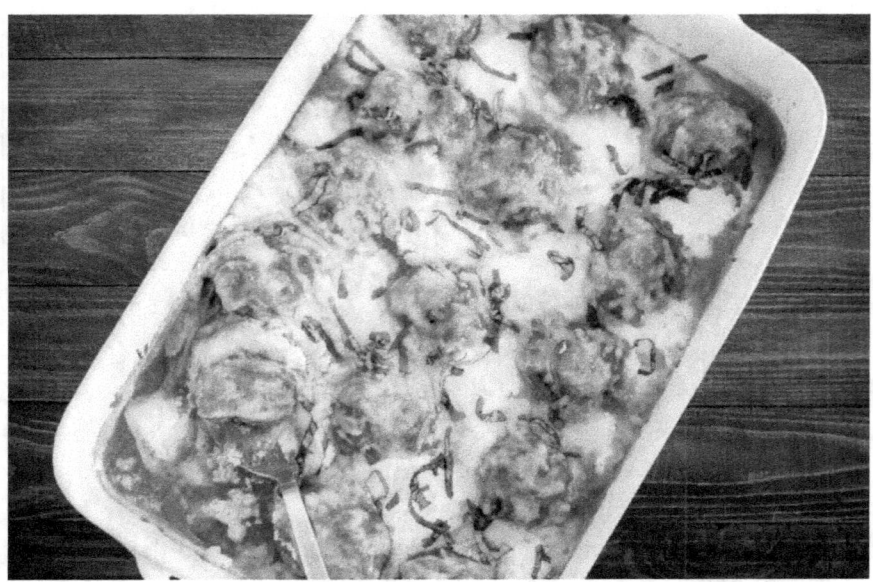

This recipe combines two classic recipes into one incredibly flavorful dish that will surely be a hit. The classic casserole is a good way to use up leftovers, and when you combine it with Italian meatballs, you get an incredibly flexible and convenient all-in-one meal.

Forming the meatballs is easy, and once you get the hang of it, you'll be making them like a pro. One helpful tip is to dip your measuring spoon into a cup of cold water between each scoop. This will help release the meat mixture from the spoon. Then, use your hands to roll the meat around to form the meatballs. I recommend using a two-tablespoon measuring spoon, so you only need one scoop per ball.

You can make the meatballs and the sauce ahead of time and throw the casserole together in just a few minutes. However, if the meatballs are cold, you will need to warm them up before you construct the casserole. This recipe will store in the fridge for about a week, or you can freeze it for up to three months.

You can also use this recipe to make traditional meatballs by cooking them in a skillet over high heat. Cook each meatball for approximately two minutes on each side to get a nice sear on the outside. They are done when they hit an internal temperature of one hundred and sixty degrees Fahrenheit.

This recipe is prime for customization. You can replace ground beef with any ground meat, like chicken, turkey, pork, Italian sausage, or a combination of these meats.

Once your casserole is done, garnish it with a basil chiffonade. *What's a chiffonade?* You may be wondering. It's when you thinly slice an herb like basil or mint. It's pleasing to the eye and releases more of the aromatic notes of the herb. This can be achieved by stacking and rolling the leaves into a tight cylinder and finely slicing them into thin strips.

Difficulty Level: 3 out of 5 Meatballs

Prep Time: 15 Minutes

Cook Time: 1 Hour

Servings: 4

Nutritional Facts:
(Per Serving)

Calories 824

Protein 57g

Fat 59g

Total Carbohydrates 12g

Meatballs:

2 pounds of ground beef

1/2 cup of parmesan cheese, grated

2 eggs

1/4 cup of onion, grated

3 garlic cloves, minced

3 tablespoons of fresh parsley, minced

1/2 teaspoon of Italian seasoning

2 teaspoons of salt

1 teaspoon of pepper

Sauce:

6 ounces of tomato paste

1/3 cup beef broth

1/4 cup parmesan cheese, grated

Toppings:

1/2 cup mozzarella cheese, shredded

1/2 cup ricotta cheese

2 to 3 tablespoons fresh basil, thinly sliced

Put all the meatball ingredients in a medium-sized bowl and mix until well combined.

Form the ground beef mixture into meatballs using approximately 2 tablespoons for each. Place meatballs on a parchment paper-lined baking sheet.

Bake the meatballs at 400°F for 20 minutes. While the meatballs are baking, prepare the sauce by combining the beef broth, parmesan cheese, and tomato paste in a small bowl. Stir until a uniform consistency is achieved, then set aside.

When the meatballs are done, place them in a casserole dish, cover them with the sauce, and top each meatball with a spoonful of ricotta cheese.

Cover it all with the mozzarella cheese and broil for 3-5 minutes or until the cheese has melted and brown spots start to appear on top.

Let cool for 5-10 minutes, garnish with basil, and enjoy!

Korean Barbeque Style Ground Beef

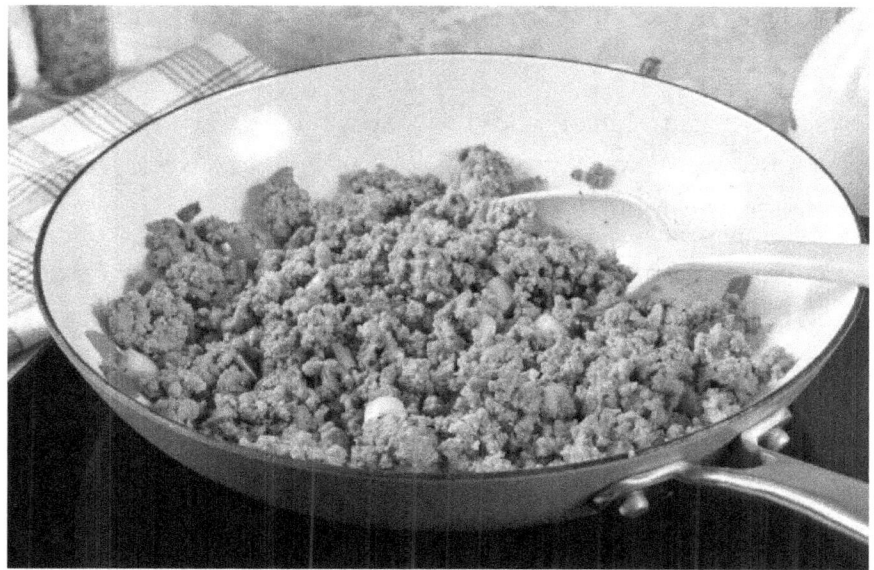

This high-protein and high-fat recipe is fast and easy, so keep it in your back pocket whenever you crave a sweet and savory dish. Best of all, it doesn't contain any added sugar.

A box grater will work for grating the ginger, but a food processor will do it in half the time. However, you must consider the clean-up time as well. When using a food processor, throw in the garlic with the ginger and pulse it until you have achieved a minced consistency. Be careful not to over-process it, or you will end up with mush.

Separating the white and green parts of green onions allows you to use them for different applications in one recipe. The whites get sautéed and add a caramelized onion note to the dish, while the greens are used as a garnish to add a sharper onion flavor.

You will know when this dish is done after most of the liquid has either been absorbed by the meat or has evaporated. This reduction of liquid concentrates the flavors and enhances the overall dining experience.

This dish can be made ahead of time and reheated on the stove or in a microwave. It will store in the fridge for up to a week and a half or in the freezer for up to three months.

You can add peas and carrots to this recipe if you like. A bag of frozen peas and carrots would work well for this addition. Ensure you defrost and add them to the dish after the ground beef is cooked. If you want to add another level of flavor, try roasting the peas and carrots in a pan or in the oven first.

Feel free to adjust the spice level of this dish to your liking. You can remove the chili garlic sauce if you dislike spicy foods or substitute it with sriracha if that's what you have. You could go buck wild and do both; it's up to you, but you may want to consider anyone's preference who you may be enjoying this dish with. You can always add more spice later.

I like to eat my Korean barbeque style ground beef in a bowl alongside some avocado with sea salt sprinkled on top, but you can also eat it over steamed jasmine rice or wrapped in a leaf of lettuce, such as romaine or butter lettuce if you wish.

This recipe was inspired by the traditional Korean dish known as bulgogi, which is very similar to this recipe. Instead of ground beef, it calls for strips of beef like top sirloin or ribeye. To make a traditional bulgogi, marinate the mea overnight, grill it, and serve it the same way you would this recipe.

Difficulty Level: 2 out of 5 Meatballs

Prep Time: 10 Minutes

Cook Time: 10 Minutes

Servings: 2

Nutritional Facts:
(Per Serving)

Calories 882

Protein 40g

Fat 68g

Total Carbohydrates 12g

1 pound of ground beef

6 cloves of garlic, minced

2 teaspoons of ginger, grated

2 tablespoons of coconut oil

1 tablespoon of toasted sesame oil

1 tablespoon of rice vinegar

2 tablespoons of coconut aminos

1 tablespoon of chili garlic sauce

1 tablespoon of Worcestershire sauce

1 bunch of green onions, washed and sliced, with the white and green parts separated

1 teaspoon black pepper

1 tablespoon of toasted sesame seeds

Melt the coconut oil in a skillet over high heat. Add the white portion of the green onions to the skillet and cook for 1 minute.

Add the garlic to the skillet and cook for 30 seconds, stirring to avoid burning. Add the ground beef to the skillet, breaking it up into small pieces with a spatula as you cook it. Cook until no longer pink.

Reduce heat to medium and add the ginger, sesame oil, coconut aminos, Worcestershire sauce, pepper, rice vinegar, and chili garlic sauce.

Continue cooking until most of the moisture is absorbed or evaporated, about 2 minutes.

Mix in 1/3 cup of the green portion of the green onions, stir to mix, and continue cooking for another minute.

Remove from heat and let cool for 5 minutes.

Garnish with green onions and toasted sesame seeds.

Serve on top of rice, inside leaf lettuce, or alone.

Ground Beef and Cheddar Scramble

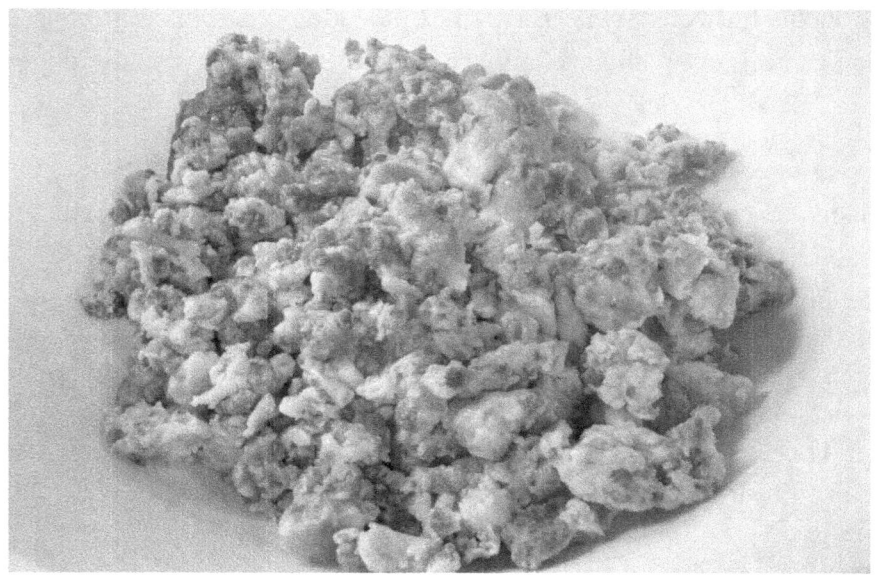

This recipe packs fifty-three grams of protein, can be enjoyed any time of day, and is highly customizable.

This recipe uses an immersion blender to make the eggs extra fluffy. If you do not have an immersion blender, you can use a whisk or a fork to scramble the eggs, but an immersion blender will do it in half the time and make the eggs super frothy, resulting in extremely fluffy eggs.

You will know the eggs are done cooking when they no longer appear watery. It's important not to overcook the eggs, or they will dry out, so as soon as they are cooked, add the cheese and remove from heat.

This dish can be stored in the fridge for one week, but it's best just after it is prepared. Re-heated eggs almost always come out dry and rubbery.

Scrambles are a great way to use up any leftovers you may have lying around. You can substitute the ground beef with steak, sausage, or bacon, but you may need to adjust the ratios. Regarding the cheese, you can mix it up and use any cheese you like. Pepper jack will give this dish a nice kick, or try using mozzarella.

Some caramelized onions would also make a great addition to this dish. You can also add a splash of milk or cream to the egg mixture to make the eggs extra fluffy, but this is not required, especially if you stay away from dairy. If that's you, try aged cheeses like parmesan, they are low in lactose and may not affect you the same way other cheeses might.

This dish can be garnished with chives, parsley, or cilantro to give it a south-of-the-border twist.

Difficulty Level: 3 out of 5 Meatballs

Prep Time: 10 Minutes

Cook Time: 10 Minutes

Servings: 2

Nutritional Facts:
(Per Serving)

Calories 760

Protein 53g

Fat 58g

Total Carbohydrates

1 pound of ground beef

4 eggs

1 ounce of cheddar cheese, shredded

2 teaspoons of salt

½ teaspoon of black pepper

Set a medium-sized skillet over high heat and add the ground beef.

Use a spatula to break up the ground beef as it cooks. Continue mixing the ground beef as it cooks; it will be done when no more pink is left.

Crack the eggs into a bowl while the ground beef is cooking and add salt and pepper. Use an immersion blender to scramble the eggs until they are frothy.

Lower the heat to medium and pour the egg mixture into the skillet. Using a spatula, continuously mix the eggs and ground beef until the eggs are cooked.

Add the cheddar cheese to the skillet and fold it in.

Place your scramble in a serving bowl, add your garnish of choice, and enjoy.

Fast Flavorful Chuck Roast

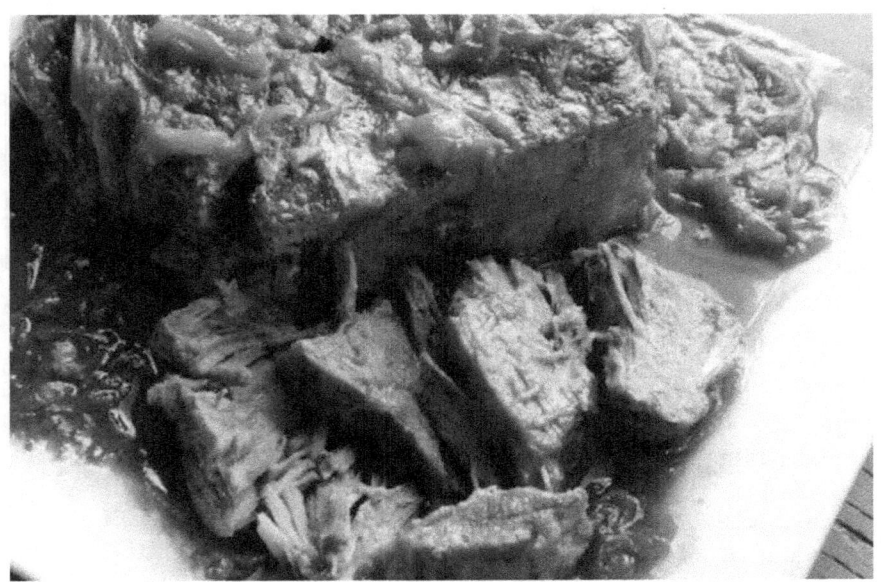

This is the perfect dish when you're short on time and need a hearty meal for the week or the whole family. The base recipe has only five ingredients and requires very little preparation, making it ideal for busy weekdays.

I love pressure cookers, which is what makes this recipe so quick to prepare! You can make this dish in a slow cooker or bake it in a Dutch oven, but a pressure cooker is the fastest way to cook a chuck roast without sacrificing flavor or texture. I use an Instant Pot but any pressure cooker will do. The best part about using a pressure cooker is that you can cook a frozen chuck roast in under two hours. It'll be just as good as if you had waited several days for it to thaw before cooking.

Most experienced home cooks may bock at this recipe for not browning the roast before braising/ pressure cooking, but I have found that taking the extra time to brown the roast is not critical and does not lessen the flavor much of this dish. If you have the time, you can brown the chuck roast on all sides on a skillet or on a barbecue grill before pressure cooking but you may need to reduce the cooking time if you do.

You can eat your chuck roast in a bowl with some of the cooking liquid or broth. It's like a stew, this way you'll get all the additional nutrients from the broth. This fast flavorful chuck roast recipe is similar to my pot roast recipe but much simpler and faster. It's ideal for anyone following a low-carb or carnivore diet.

I make this recipe at least once a week and divide it into portions for meal preparation. These can be frozen for up to three months or stored in the fridge for up to a week. I recommend reheating the chuck roast in the cooking liquid so the meat doesn't dry out. You can do this in the microwave or on the stove. The cooking liquid can also be used to cook anything else you want to impart additional flavor to.

Like all of my recipes, I encourage you to experiment and make them your own. You could try omitting the beef broth and Worcestershire sauce for this recipe. Only using the coconut aminos as a cooking liquid gives this dish a unique flavor that is hard to describe but hits hard on the umami scale. You can also try reducing the cooking liquid to create a more flavorful broth. If you do this, remove the chuck roast and the onions first and set your instant pot on sauté mode for thirty minutes to an hour with the lid off.

I like using coconut aminos instead of soy sauce to avoid the potential hormonal effects that can arise from consuming too much soy. Soy is in many products, and I try to avoid it when I can. Coconut aminos are also gluten-free! *What are coconut aminos?* It's made from the fermented sap of coconut palms and have slightly sweet and savory notes.

I included Worcestershire sauce in this recipe to add an additional layer of flavor to the dish. It's inexpensive, stores in your pantry for a long time, and a little goes a long way.

Difficulty Level: 3 out of 5 Meatballs

Prep Time: 5 Minutes

Cook Time: 1 Hour

Servings: 6

Nutritional Facts:
(Per Serving)
Calories 562
Protein 58g
Fat 34g
Total Carbohydrates

3-5 pounds of chuck roast

1 cup of beef broth

1/2 of a yellow onion, peeled and sliced into 1-inch thick rings

1/4 cup of coconut aminos

1 tablespoon of Worcestershire sauce

Combine the beef broth, coconut aminos, and the Worcestershire sauce in the instant pot and stir to mix. Arrange onion slices in a single layer on the bottom of the instant pot.

Place the chuck roast on top of the onions. Place the lid on the pot and ensure the pressure relief valve is in the closed position.

Cooking times:

Defrosted: Pressure cook on high for 45 minutes and let the pressure naturally release for 15 minutes.

Frozen: Pressure cook on high for 1 hour and let the pressure naturally release for 20 minutes.

Carefully open the pressure relief valve to relieve any residual pressure. Remove the roast from the pot and let it rest for 10 minutes.

Hand shred or rough chop the chuck roast, serve in a bowl with some of the broth, and enjoy!

Texas-Style Smoked Brisket

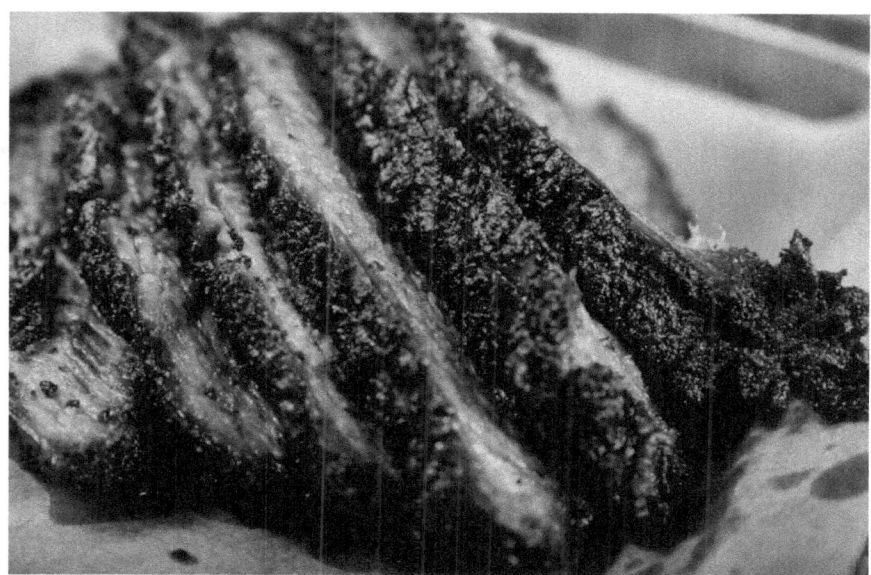

I have always enjoyed Texas-style barbeque, but a recent trip to Austin, Texas, revealed its true potential. I have been smoking brisket for years, but my trip to Austin inspired me to take my brisket game to the next level, and this recipe is a result of that.

To make this recipe properly, you will need a smoker, butcher paper, a meat thermometer, oak and mesquite lump charcoal, and a spray bottle.

Brisket comes from the chest of a cow and is one of the nine primal cuts of beef. A whole brisket is called a packer and is composed of two muscles, the point and the flat. Most grocery stores sell the flat, which is leaner and is where traditional sliced brisket comes from. It's also commonly used to make pastrami. The point is where the fat is at, and it's highly marbled and full of flavor. Some people choose to separate the point and the flat and cook them separately, but I like to cook them as one. The fat from the point helps to keep the flat moist, and I love seeing that massive cut of meat in the smoker, but there is nothing wrong with separating them. If you choose this path, you will have shorter cooking times, and each portion will cook more evenly.

Whether you get a point, a flat, or a whole-packer brisket, you will inevitably need to trim your brisket. This is a relatively simple process of removing excessive fat and cutting off thinner portions to ensure even cooking. You will want to do this when the meat is cold; the warmer it gets, the softer the fat will be, making it more challenging to trim. You will want to remove all the hard fat, but you can Leave approximately one-quarter to one-third of an inch of the soft fat all the way around. This will help keep your brisket from drying out. You can also trim the thinner edges as these may dry out during cooking. Keep your trimmings to make ground beef or as a special treat for your k9 companions.

Now, you have a choice: to brine or not to brine. A brine is a saltwater solution with added herbs and spices that will impart additional flavor and moisture to your end product. This is optional, and most barbeque restaurants skip this step. If you choose to brine your brisket, you will need a large container, especially if you use a whole brisket. I have included a brine recipe and instructions following the brisket recipe.

Use mustard as a binder to help create that famous bark or crust. You can use whatever seasoning you like. I prefer Montreal steak seasoning, and the world-famous Terry Black's in Austin, Texas, uses good old Lowry's seasoning salt. Whatever seasoning you choose, make sure to get a healthy layer of it on all sides of your brisket. This is a thick cut, so you can go heavy on the seasoning to ensure there is enough to flavor it all the way through.

My preferred type of smoker is the offset smoker. I use mesquite lump charcoal as the base of the fire and a propane torch to light it. Once the charcoal gets going, place a small chunk of oak on top of the coals to produce the smoke. If it stops smoking, hit it with a spray of your apple cider vinegar solution, and it should smoke right up.

I prefer oak, but you can use hickory or any other hardwood. The type of wood you use will impart its unique flavor onto the meat, so feel free to experiment with different types or multiple types of hardwood to get a unique flavor profile.

You can adjust the temperature once your smoker gets going by opening and closing the dampeners. There is usually one on the smoke stack and one on the inlet of the firebox. By adjusting the dampeners, you change the airflow, which reduces or increases the temperature of the smoker. You will want to keep your smoker right around 250°F during the smoking process. You must monitor and experiment with the dampeners to achieve the correct temperature throughout the smoking process.

Before you place the brisket in your smoker, ensure the grates are clean. Then, place a metal bowl or pan near the firebox and fill it with a fifty-fifty mixture of water and apple cider vinegar. This will ensure a moist environment inside the smoking chamber, helping to keep your brisket from drying out.

Add charcoal and the hardwood of your choosing as needed throughout the smoking process. I recommend checking on it at a minimum every hour. This is also an excellent time to mist your brisket and top off the bowl with the apple cider vinegar mixture.

You can complete the cooking process in the smoker if you like. However, this uses a lot of charcoal and requires constant tending to keep the fire going. I like to finish my brisket in a two-hundred-degree oven. Either way, after about four hours of smoking, you should have a very dark-colored bark, and this is what you want. Now it's time to wrap your brisket in two layers of unbleached and un-waxed butcher paper or aluminum foil and bake or continue smoking it at two hundred and fifty degrees Fahrenheit. Spritz your brisket again with the apple cider vinegar mixture before you wrap it. Seal it up tight by wrapping it once, then place the edge of the paper in the middle of the second one to create a good seal. Place the seam side down to hold the paper in place.

After four hours, check the brisket's temperature to ensure it's done using a meat thermometer. It should be one hundred and ninety-five degrees Fahrenheit in the middle. Then, leave it wrapped and let it rest for at least thirty minutes to one hour to let the juices redistribute throughout the meat.

Slice and serve with mac and cheese and sautéed greens, or use some homemade sourdough garlic bread and coleslaw to make the best sandwich you've ever had. This brisket is also wonderful on it's own and this is how I enjoy it.

Difficulty Level: 5 out of 5 Meatballs

Prep Time: 10 Minutes

Cook Time: 8 Hours

Servings: 12

Nutritional Facts:
(Per Serving)

Calories 595

Protein 78g

Fat 28g

Total Carbohydrates >1g

10 pounds of brisket

2 tablespoons of yellow mustard

2 tablespoons of stone ground mustard

2 tablespoons of Montreal steak seasoning

2 cup of apple cider vinegar

2 cup of water, filtered

Trim excess fat and thinner portions of the brisket.

Optional: Brine your brisket overnight

Dry off your brisket well with a paper towel. Allow your brisket to come to room temperature for at least one hour before putting it in the smoker.

Get the smoker going and place a metal bowl or pan of half water and half apple cider vinegar in the smoker to retain moisture.

Mix the mustards in a small bowl and spread a thin layer on all sides of the brisket. Liberally season the brisket with the Montreal steak seasoning on all sides.

Place the brisket on the smoker with the fat side up, adjust the dampeners, and smoke for 4 hours at 250°F.

Check your fire, add more wood and charcoal as needed, and spray the brisket with the apple cider vinegar mixture after the first hour and every hour thereafter throughout the smoking process.

Preheat your oven to 250°F Remove the brisket from the smoker, wrap it in two layers of butcher paper, and bake at 250°F for another 4 hours or until an internal temperature of 195°F is reached.

Let your brisket rest for 30 minutes to one hour, then slice against the grain and enjoy!

Brine Recipe

Using a brine can add additional moisture and add additional layers of flavor to briskets, turkey, and many other meats. It's not required, but it will make for a juicier and more flavorful end product.

Difficulty Level: 1 out of 5 Meatballs

Prep Time: 5 Minutes

Cook Time: None

Servings: 1

1/2 cup of salt

1/2 cup of coconut aminos

5 cloves of garlic

1 large white onion

5 bay leaves

1 tablespoon peppercorns

Filtered water

Add all of the ingredients to a bucket or another container large enough to hold the brisket and stir to mix.

After you trim your brisket, place it in the brine solution.

Cover and store in the fridge overnight.

Burnt Ends

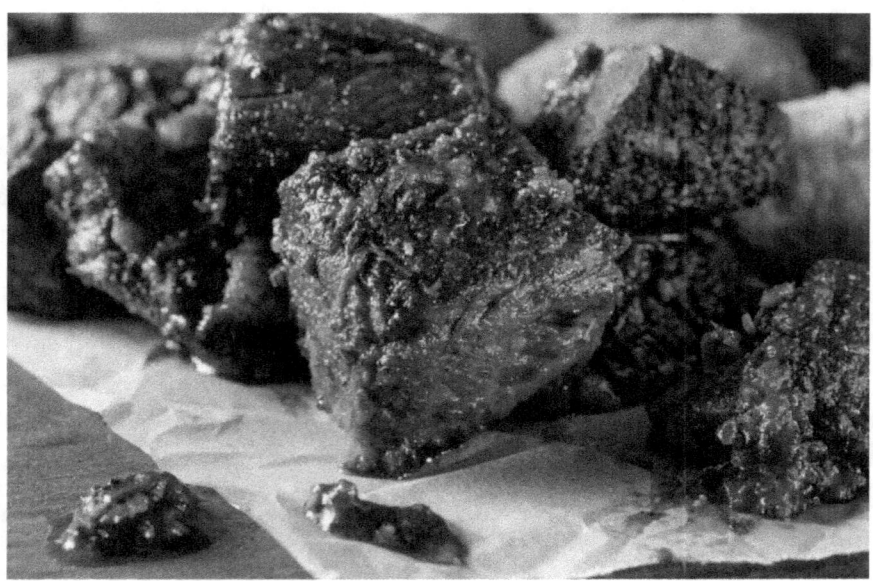

These meaty morsels will melt in your mouth and keep your coming back for more. Burnt ends are traditionally made with the point or fatty end of a brisket but this recipe calls for chuck roast instead. A brisket can be expensive and a little intimidating since it is such a big cut of meat but a chuck roast is smaller making it easier to manage. It's also more economical and makes for wonderfully tender and delicious burnt ends.

To do it right, you will need a smoker, but you could impart some smoke flavor by using the foil pack method on a gas grill. Oak is my go-to wood for smoking beef, but you can use whatever hardwood you prefer. Hickory is also a great choice and will add a complementary flavor to this dish.

You can read more on smoking meat in the Basic Cooking Methods chapter on page 25 or in my Texas-Style Smoked Brisket recipe on page 81.

Smoke the burnt ends for longer if you like more smoke flavor. When you're done smoking them, add the sauce, cover the pan very tightly to retain the moisture, and continue cooking at two hundred and fifty degrees Fahrenheit for two to four hours to allow the connective tissues to breakdown and create that decadent juiciness you want in burnt ends. You will know when the burnt ends are done when you squeeze one between your fingers, and it breaks apart easily.

Burnt ends can be made in advance by smoking them ahead of time. Let them cool and store them in the fridge. When you're ready to finish them, place them in the oven at two hundred and fifty degrees Fahrenheit for one hour, and bam you have tender and juicy burnt ends. These finished burnt ends can be stored in the fridge for up to a week or frozen for up to three months.

If you want to change the flavor of this recipe, you can try using different seasonings like Lowry's seasoning salt or even a basic salt and pepper. Remember you are the one who will be enjoying this dish so make it your own and try new and unique flavors to find what you like.

Difficulty Level: 4 out of 5 Meatballs

Prep Time: 10 Minutes

Cook Time: 4 Hours

Servings: 6

Nutritional Facts:
(Per Serving)

Calories 440

Protein 44g

Fat 26g

Total Carbohydrates

3-5 pound chuck roast

1 tablespoon of stone ground mustard

1 tablespoon of yellow mustard

2 tablespoons of Montreal steak seasoning

1/4 cup of apple cider vinegar

1/4 cup of filtered water

1/4 cup of beef broth

1 tablespoon of Worcestershire sauce

1/4 cup barbecue sauce

Preheat your smoker to 250°F.

Combine the water and apple cider vinegar in a spray bottle.

Cut the chuck roast into 1 1/2-inch pieces.

Place the pieces of chuck roast in a large bowl. Combine both types of mustard and mix, then toss with the chuck roast to coat each piece. Add the Montreal steak seasoning, then mix to coat each piece with seasoning evenly. Place the prepared chuck roast in a half-sized foil pan.

When your smoker is to temperature, place the pan in the smoker and let them smoke for 1 hour.

After 1 hour tend the fire and add more wood and charcoal as needed, flip the burnt ends over and spray them with the apple cider vinegar mixture. Continue to smoke them for another hour.

Preheat oven to 250°F.

Remove the smoked ends from the smoker and spray them again with the apple cider vinegar mixture. Mix the beef broth, Worcestershire sauce, and BBQ sauce with the chuck roast.

Cover the foil pan with more foil to create a tight seal and bake at 250°F for 2-4 hours or until an internal temperature of 195°F achieved.

Remove from the oven, allow to rest for 10 minutes, then enjoy!

Cheeseburger Casserole

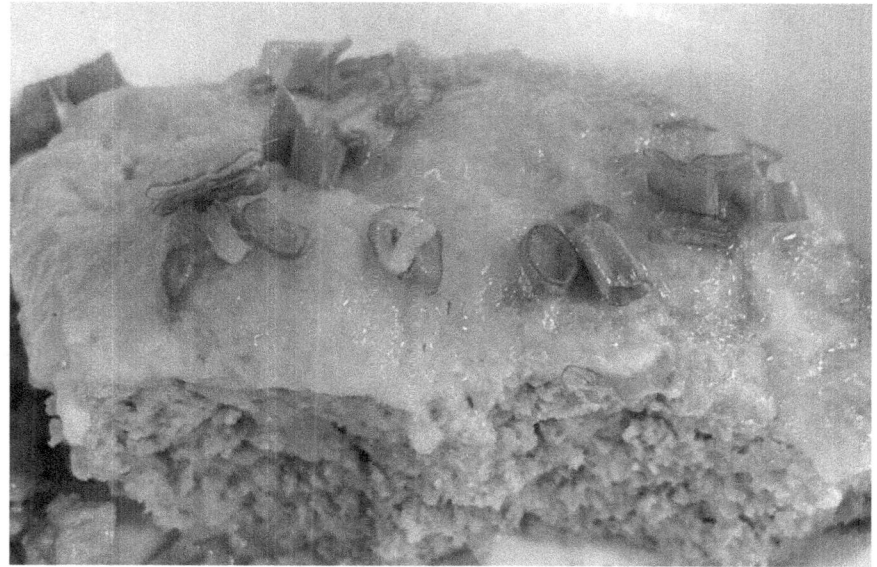

This cheeseburger casserole recipe is easy to make, delicious, and will fuel your body for hours on end.

Casseroles have been a staple in kitchens around the world for centuries, evolving from simple one-pot meals to elaborate dishes enjoyed at family gatherings and potlucks. The term "casserole" originally referred to the pan used to cook the dish, deriving from the French word "casse," meaning "box." Early casseroles often combined rice or pasta with meats and vegetables, creating a hearty meal in a single dish.

Casseroles gained popularity in the United States during the 20th century, especially during the Great Depression and World War II, when home cooks sought to stretch ingredients and create nourishing meals with minimal waste. The convenience and versatility of casseroles made them a go-to for busy families. The post-war era saw an explosion of casserole recipes, often featuring canned soups and other convenient ingredients, which were heavily promoted by food companies.

The cheeseburger casserole is a relatively modern creation that combines the classic flavors of a cheeseburger in a comforting, low-carb dish. This recipe is perfect for ketogenic or carnivore diets.

Most ovens have a broil setting, and if yours doesn't, check your toaster oven, as it may have one. This setting completes the dish by melting and browning the cheese, which adds flavor and makes the casserole look more appealing. You could use a kitchen torch to melt and brown the cheese in a pinch, but be careful not to burn yourself.

If you are making this dish ahead of time, stop after the casserole's initial baking. Then, when you are ready to eat, microwave your portion for a minute and then continue following the steps to melt the cheese on top. This dish will store in the fridge for up to a week or for up to 3 months in the freezer.

Depending on your preferences, you can add a variety of spices to the ground beef mixture to enhance the flavor of this dish, such as taco seasoning, garlic powder, or smoked paprika for a little kick.

Eating this dish with a side of shredded lettuce, onions, tomatoes, and pickles will give you a more cheeseburger like experience and if you throw some bacon up on that, you'll have a bacon cheeseburger casserole. I recommend pairing this recipe with my Bacon Twists recipe found on page 149. You could also add bread or cornflake crumbs on top of the casserole just before you melt the cheese for a bit of a crunch, but to keep it low-carb, replace the bread crumbs with pork rind crumbs, also known as pork panko.

Difficulty Level: 2 out of 5 Meatballs

Prep Time: 5 Minutes

Cook Time: 45 Minutes

Servings: 4

Nutritional Facts:
(Per Serving)

Calories 788

Protein 53g

Fat 61g

Total Carbohydrates

6 eggs

2 teaspoons of salt

2 pounds of ground beef

4 ounces of mild cheddar cheese, shredded

2 green onions, washed and thinly sliced

Preheat oven to 350°F.

Combine eggs and salt in a medium-sized bowl and mix to scramble the eggs.

Add the ground beef and mix with the egg mixture until combined.

Grease a baking dish or cast iron skillet and add the ground beef mixture. Level out the mixture with a spatula.

Bake at 350°F for 45 minutes.

Remove the casserole from the oven and preheat the broiler to high.

Spread the cheese evenly on top of the casserole and place under the broiler for 3-5 minutes or until the cheese is melted and starts to brown.

Carefully remove the casserole from the broiler and let it cool for 5 minutes.

Garnish with green onions, and enjoy!

CHICKEN

Chicken is one of the most versatile and widely available proteins, making it a staple in many kitchens—and for good reason. In this chapter, you'll find various recipes featuring chicken in all its forms, from crispy wings to a comforting chicken bone broth. Whether you prefer it roasted, grilled, shredded, or pan-fried in butter, chicken offers endless possibilities.

Chicken is unique in that they offer two kinds of meat: white and dark. White meat, which comes from the breast, is lean and delicate. It's great for lighter dishes but can dry out quickly if overcooked. On the other hand, dark meat, found in the legs, thighs, and wings, boasts a richer flavor thanks to its higher fat content, which also helps to keep it tender and juicy. Some recipes in this chapter call for specific cuts to capture the right balance of texture and taste, but in many cases, you can substitute cuts based on your preference or what you have on hand.

Whenever possible, I recommend using chicken with the skin on—not just for the added flavor and crispiness but also for the valuable nutrients contained in the fat. Fat is a fantastic fuel for your body and helps you stay fuller longer. It also adds richness to dishes, especially when rendered into sauces and broths.

Chicken's subtle flavor lends it to easily take on bold marinades, subtle herbs, or even simple salt and pepper. In this chapter, I encourage you to explore its many possibilities, whether crafting a slow-cooked stew or throwing together a quick weeknight meal. Chicken is an essential part of the Protein Lifestyle because it offers variety, nourishment, and flexibility.

Creamy Buffalo Chicken Wrap

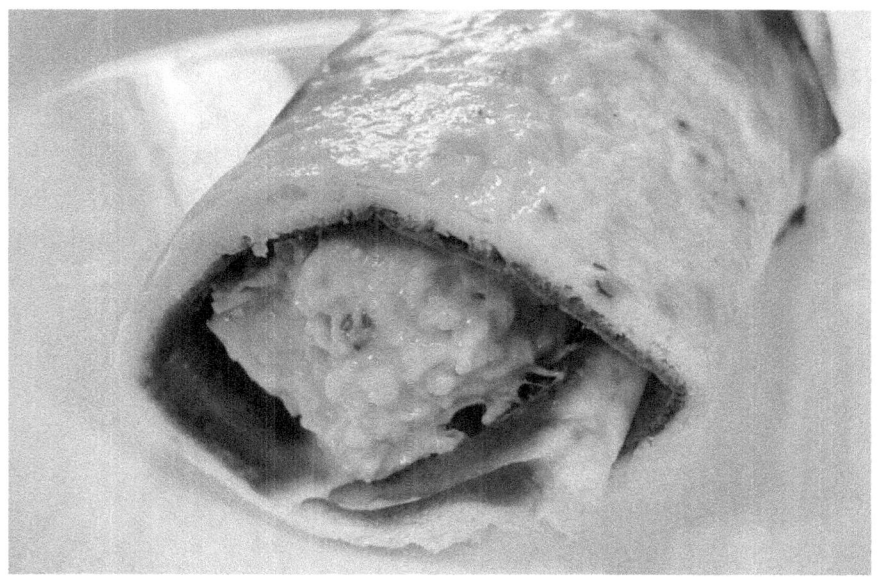

The Creamy Buffalo Chicken Wrap is so good you won't miss the carbs. I love this recipe because it's versatile, low-carb, and so delicious that you'll want to eat it daily. If you dislike spice, you could substitute my ranch dip recipe on page 159 for the buffalo sauce to make a cool ranch wrap.

You can use whatever kind of buffalo sauce you want, but I love the Primal Kitchen buffalo sauce; it tastes great, is made with avocado oil, and has no artificial ingredients. You could also use rotisserie or boiled chicken.

When I say this recipe is versatile, I mean it. You could eat the chicken mixture on its own like chicken salad, in a wrap, or use it as a dip.

Difficulty Level: 1 out of 5 Meatballs

Prep Time: 10 Minutes

Cook Time: 2 Minutes

Servings: 2

Nutritional Facts:
(Per Serving)

Calories 314

Protein 44g

Fat 13g

Total Carbohydrates

1 (12.5) ounce can of chicken breast

1/4 cup of cottage cheese

1/4 cup of cheddar cheese, shredded

2 tablespoons of buffalo sauce

1 tablespoon of cream cheese

1 bunch of green onions, washed and sliced thinly

Drain the liquid from the canned chicken and add it to a medium-sized microwave-safe bowl.

Add the cottage cheese, shredded cheese, cream cheese, and buffalo sauce to the bowl.

Mash and mix everything together with a fork until a uniform consistency is achieved.

Microwave for 1 minute and then stir and microwave for 1 more minute or until the cheese is melted.

Add 2 tablespoons of the sliced green onions to the bowl and mix.

Use this creamy buffalo chicken in a wrap, or enjoy it as is.

Cottage Cheese Wrap

This recipe, is a game changer for anyone following a ketogenic or carnivore diet. It is very low in carbohydrates and can be used instead of tortillas for tacos, burritos, and wraps.

If you don't use the wrap right away, it will get hard, but you can soften it up by microwaving it for 20-30 seconds, and it will become pliable again.

Difficulty Level: 2 out of 5 Meatballs

Prep Time: 10 Minutes

Cook Time: 2 Hours

Servings: 2

Nutritional Facts:
(Per Serving)

Calories 193

Protein 19g

Fat 10g

Total Carbohydrates

8 ounces of cottage cheese

2 eggs

2 tablespoons of parmesan cheese

Pepper to taste

Preheat oven to 350°F. Combine all ingredients in a blender. Blend on medium until the mixture is smooth.

Pour the mixture onto a half-size baking sheet lined with parchment paper. Use a rubber spatula to spread the mixture evenly across the parchment paper.

Bake at 350°F for 30 to 45 minutes or until the top starts to brown. Remove the wrap from the oven and let it cool for 3 minutes.

Cut the wrap in half and use them like you would a tortilla.

Bone Broth

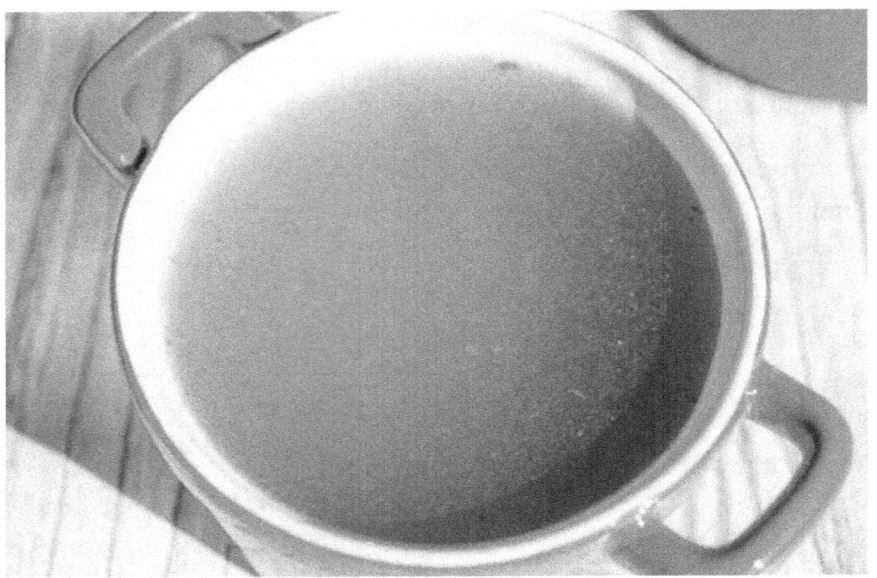

This simple and delicious bone broth recipe can be used as a base for soups and sauces or enjoyed alone. It's also the perfect remedy for a cold or upset stomach.

Bone broths have been a staple in traditional cooking for thousands of years, and they're a fantastic way to use parts of the animal that would otherwise go to waste.

This recipe was initially designed to provide relief for anyone suffering from digestive disorders like IBS, IBD, Crohn's, or ulcerative colitis. Ginger is included in this recipe as it soothes the gut. The collagen and gelatin from the bones can help heal the lining of the digestive tract and do wonders for your skin, hair, and nails.

This recipe offers the option to make chicken or beef bone broth, but it does not contain all of the traditional ingredients due to the FODMAPs or fermentable sugars in them. If you want more flavor and are unaffected by FODMAPs, add pepper, garlic, celery, and onions to this recipe.

You have a few options when choosing the type of bones for this recipe. Beef bones from deboned roasts from your butcher are perfect, but you can also use beef shanks as called for in the recipe. You can use the carcass leftover from a rotisserie chicken or chicken legs for chicken bones. You can even include some chicken feet if you want even more collagen.

If you have an upset stomach, IBS, or any other bowel disorder, you should remove the fat during a flare-up as it is harder to digest. You can do this by refrigerating the broth overnight and then removing the solidified fat layer that forms on top. If you do not have IBS or another good reason to remove the fat, I highly recommend you keep it. Your body needs this vital macronutrient to function properly.

This recipe does not require any special equipment. A pressure cooker like an instant pot will make the process much faster, but it can also be made in a stock pot over the stove.

The lemon rind will add a bitter note to the broth, so to avoid this, the recipe calls only for the juice and zest of the lemon. Use a zester or a box grater to zest the lemon, stopping when you get to the white part of the lemon rind. If you don't have anything to zest the lemon, you can skip it and use the juice alone.

This recipe is easy to prepare because all ingredients will be strained after cooking, so everything only needs to be washed well and roughly chopped. If you use bones with meat on them, like chicken legs, you can remove the meat after cooking and use it in other recipes, like my protein pizza crust on page 112.

Bone broth can be stored in your refrigerator for up to one week or in your freezer for up to three months. I like to freeze my broth in smaller portions. This way, you can defrost only as much as you need and it will defrost faster.

Difficulty Level: 2 out of 5 Meatballs

Prep Time: 10 Minutes

Cook Time: 2 Hours

Servings: 6

4 pounds of chicken legs or beef shank or 2 pounds of bones alone

3 large carrots, washed, ends removed, and roughly chopped

2 inches of ginger, washed and roughly chopped

1 lemon, washed

1 bunch of cilantro, washed

2 tablespoons of apple cider vinegar

2 tablespoons of sea salt

Filtered water

Use a zester to remove the zest from the lemon. Cut the lemon in half, squeeze the juice, and discard the rind. Place the lemon juice and zest into a large stock pot or a 6-quart or larger pressure cooker, like an instant pot. Add the rest of the ingredients to the pot.

Cook the broth:

Pressure cooker: Pressure cook on high for 2 hours, then let the pressure naturally release for 20 minutes.

Stock Pot: Cook over high heat until the water starts to boil, then reduce to medium heat, cover, and let simmer for 4 hours.

Carefully strain your broth with a metal colander into another pot, let cool for 15 minutes and enjoy.

Zesty Lemon Pepper Wings

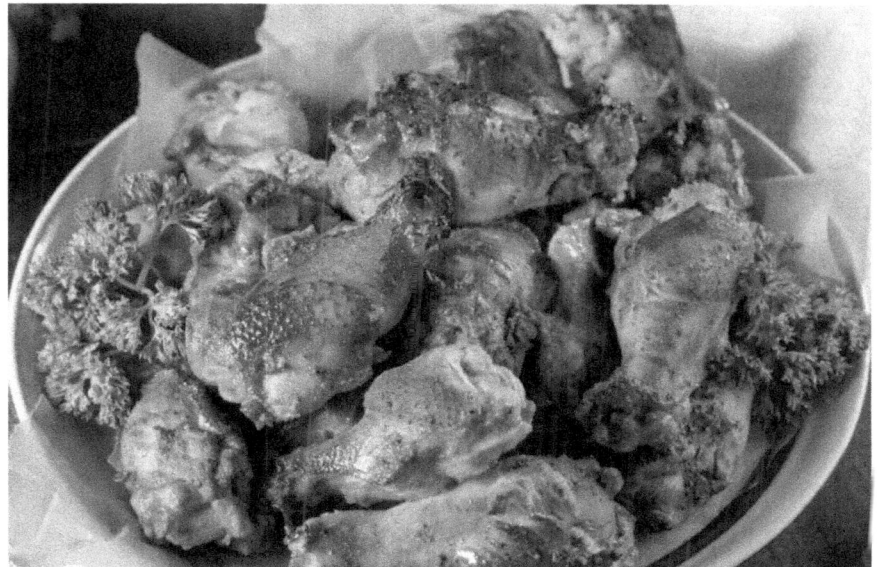

This recipe is exactly what you need to make crispy wings at home, and when you pair them with my cottage cheese ranch or blue cheese dips found on page 159, you'll never eat overpriced wings again.

Chicken wings are traditionally deep-fried, but this recipe has been crafted to make them at home in an oven or an air fryer. Cooking the wings this way helps to reduce the amount of cooking oil absorbed by the wings, and it's easier and safer because you won't have to deal with scalding hot oil.

One of the best parts about making wings at home is choosing what oil to use or, more importantly, not use. Avoid ultra-processed seed oils like corn, soy, and other vegetable oils. These oils are harmful to your health and are commonly used at many restaurants due to their affordability and availability.

Paring the type of oil and the seasonings you use will provide a plethora of flavor combinations for you to explore. This recipe calls for olive oil, but you can also use avocado oil for a more neutral flavor.

You can also use coconut oil for Asian-inspired wings. This recipe keeps it simple so you can master the technique, but once you do, you can experiment with all kinds of fun combinations, like coconut oil with garlic and ginger. You can also try salt, pepper, smoked paprika, or garlic and parmesan.

You can also sauce your wings after cooking them. In this case, you only want to season them with basic seasonings like salt and pepper. After cooking, place the wings in a large bowl and toss them in your favorite buffalo sauce or whatever sauce you like. I prefer Paleo Valley brand buffalo sauce.

When your wings are done, they should look golden brown. If your wings lack color or crispiness, place half of them back in the air fryer for a few minutes or on the top rack of your oven set to broil on high for a few minutes. Removing half of the wings will allow for less crowding and better browning.

Your wings can be stored in the fridge for about a week. When you reheat them, do it under a broiler or in an air fryer to re-crisp them.

If your wings are frozen, you can defrost them quickly by placing them in an air fryer for four minutes at four hundred degrees Fahrenheit. Drain the water from the bottom of the air fryer basket and follow the recipe as usual.

Wings can be served with carrot and or celery sticks if you wish.

Difficulty Level: 3 out of 5 Meatballs

Prep Time: 5 Minutes

Cook Time: 30 Minutes

Servings: 2

Nutritional Facts:
(Per Serving)

Calories 930

Protein 71g

Fat 68g

Total Carbohydrates

16 chicken wings

1 tablespoon of olive oil

2 tablespoons of lemon pepper seasoning

Preheat the air fryer to 450°F or the oven to 400°F.

Pat dry the wings with a paper towel and place them in a large bowl. Add the olive oil and toss to coat.

Sprinkle the lemon pepper seasoning onto the wings and toss them in the bowl to distribute the seasoning evenly.

Place wings in a single layer with room between each into the air fryer basket or a baking sheet.

Cooking the wings:

Air fryer: Air fry the wings for 8 minutes, then flip the wings over and cook for another 8 minutes or until the skin is crispy.

Oven: Bake the wings for 15 minutes, then flip the wings over and bake for another 10 minutes.

Let cool for 3-5 minutes and enjoy!

Pork Panko Crusted Chicken with Lemon Butter Drizzle

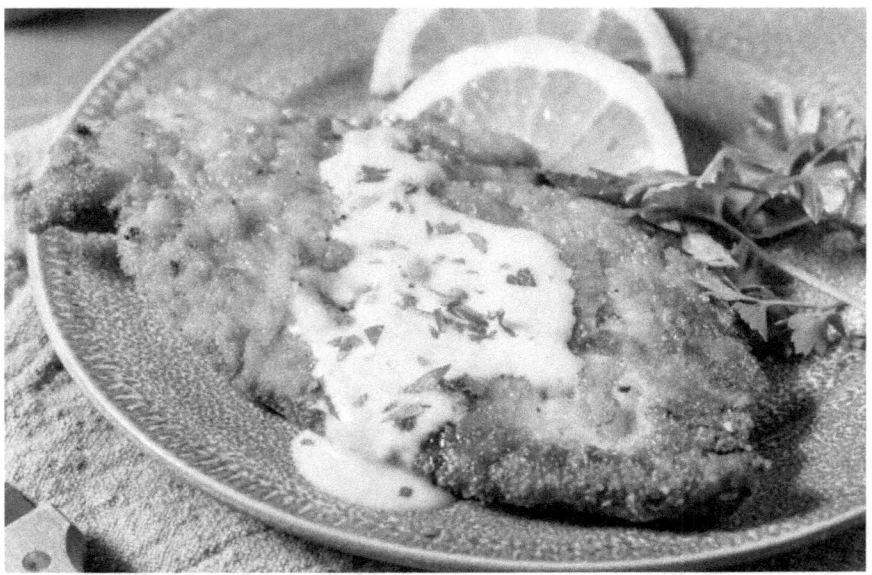

This recipe is one of the easiest and most impressive recipes in this cookbook. It was inspired by Julia Child's chicken breast meuniere: sautéed in butter found in *The Way To Cook*, but I have substituted the flour for pork panko to lower the amount of carbohydrates in this recipe.

Julia recommends accompanying this dish with baked tomatoes and fresh buttered spinach or broccoli. She states, "Sautéed potatoes would also be welcome, as would a light red wine like a Pinot Noir or Beaujolais." That sounds good to me, but I enjoy this dish solo.

This recipe calls for clarified butter, so I have included a recipe for that as an accompanying recipe for this dish.

This recipe is simple yet elegant. If you are unfamiliar with breading, I'll explain. All you need to do is spread your pork panko on a plate, press both sides of each breast into it, and then shake off any excess. Do this just before pan-frying so the pork panko doesn't get soggy.

When it comes to the chicken breasts, you can butterfly them or pound them out as directed in this recipe. You can also buy chicken breasts that the butcher has butterflied, but they can cost more, and they're easy to prepare yourself. These may also be labeled chicken milanesa in areas with a strong Hispanic presence. To butterfly a chicken breast, place your hand on top of it and, starting at the thick side of the breast, slice it in half, leaving a half inch or so at the back. Now open it up, and you're done.

Pounding out chicken breasts is also very easy. All you need to do is hit the thicker side of the breasts with a meat hammer or use your palm to hit the flat side of your chef's knife against the chicken and the cutting board. Do this in a bag or between parchment paper to reduce the mess factor.

This dish will store in the fridge for about one week but is best served fresh. You can, however, reheat it in an air fryer for best results. If you want to add another level of deliciousness to this recipe, garnish it with capers and parsley.

Difficulty Level: 3 out of 5 Meatballs

Prep Time: 5 Minutes

Cook Time: 8 Minutes

Servings: 2

Nutritional Facts:
(Per Serving)

Calories 575

Protein 57g

Fat 36g

Total Carbohydrates

4 boneless and skinless chicken breasts

Salt and pepper to taste

1 cup of pork panko

2 to 3 tablespoons of clarified butter

2 tablespoons of butter

½ of a lemon

2 tablespoons of fresh parsley, minced

Flatten the thick end of each chicken breast with a meat hammer or the flat side of your chef's knife. Strive for an even thickness throughout.

Season the breasts lightly with salt and pepper.

Just before cooking, bread them in pork panko and shake off any excess.

Set a frying pan over high heat, add the clarified butter, and, when the pan is very hot but not burning, lay in the chicken breasts one or two at a time.

Pan-fry each breast for 1-2 minutes on each side and place on a warm plate.

Wipe out the frying pan, add 2 tablespoons of butter, and heat until it turns light brown.

Squeeze a few drops of lemon juice over the chicken, pour on the hot butter, garnish with parsley, and serve at once.

Clarified Butter

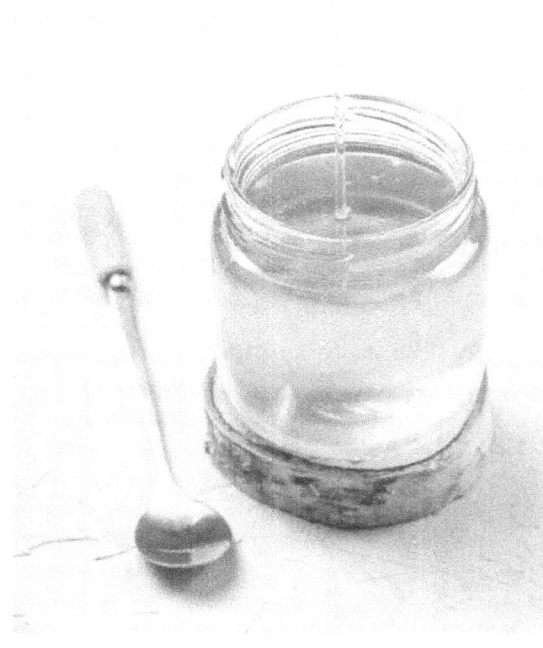

Butter is a fantastic ingredient but can be problematic for cooking because it contains milk proteins that burn at two hundred and fifty degrees Fahrenheit. Not so good for high-heat cooking, but we can overcome this by clarifying the butter.

When you clarify butter, you separate the milk solids and whey. This raises the smoke point to four hundred and fifty degrees Fahrenheit. This process also removes the moisture, allowing you to keep your clarified butter in the fridge for a year and up to six months at room temperature.

It's similar to ghee and uses the same process, but to make ghee, you don't remove the milk solids. You caramelize them. This differentiates ghee from clarified butter and gives it that well-known nutty flavor.

When you melt the butter, the milk solids and whey will separate, and after you let it sit for an hour, they will settle to the bottom.

You can use a cheesecloth to strain the butter through if you're worried about getting the milk solids in the final product, but this is not required as long as you pour it slowly.

Your clarified butter should be clear and will solidify slightly if kept at room temperature.

A fast and easy way to make clarified butter is to microwave a stick of butter in a glass or ceramic container. I like to use a Pyrex measuring cup with a pour spout to avoid making a mess.

Microwave the butter for a minute and check if it is melted. If not, microwave it for thirty-second intervals until completely melted. Be careful not to overdo it, or it can make a mess. Once melted, let it rest for about five minutes, allowing the butter solids to settle to the bottom. Now, slowly pour the butter into another vessel, making sure not to pour out the white milk solids that have settled to the bottom.

Now that you have clarified butter, you can use it to cook anything you like at high heat. I like to brown the leftover milk solids in a sauté pan and pour them over a freshly grilled steak. If you have not had steak with browned butter, you're in for a real treat.

Difficulty Level: 2 out of 5 Meatballs

Prep Time: 1 Minute

Cook Time: 10-15 Minutes

1 stick of butter

Place the butter in a saucepan over low heat.

Let the butter melt and do not stir it.

Once melted, let the butter sit for 1 hour.

Use a ladle to gently remove any foam that from the top of the butter.

Slowly pour the butter into another container, careful not to pour the milk solids that have settled on the bottom.

Use your clarified butter to cook as you would any other cooking oil.

Chicken Crust, Bacon and Beef Pizza Perfection

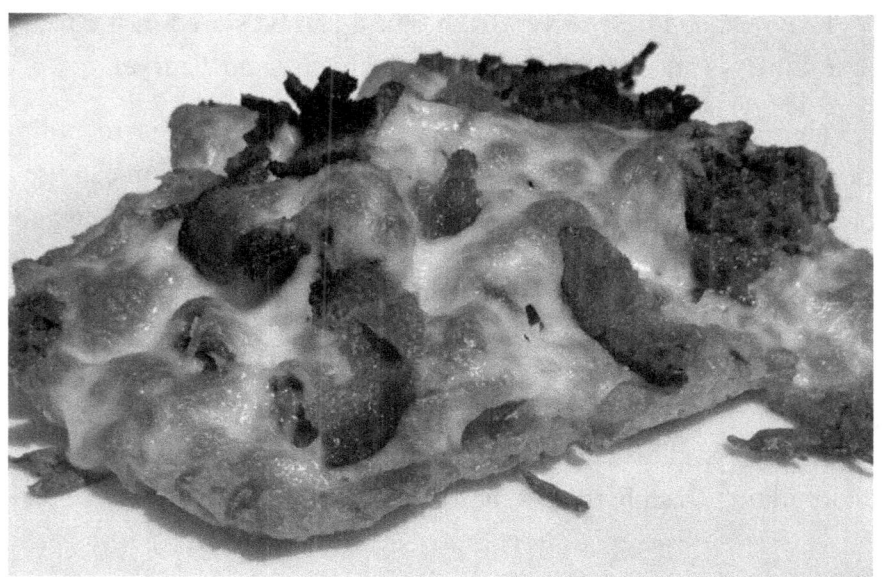

This recipe is a special treat you won't feel guilty about after consuming. When made with the accompanying chicken-based pizza crust, this recipe has just under sixty grams of protein and only two grams of carbohydrates per serving, making it a great choice when eating low-carb.

Pizza has been a staple of American cuisine since it became popular in the 1950s and 60s, and it's no wonder why. It's delicious, and the variety of toppings you can add makes it a popular dish with the whole family.

I have included a five-minute preparation time for this recipe because if you make the crust, bacon, and ground beef ahead, it only takes a few minutes to prepare up this savory dish. If you don't prep ahead, it may take thirty to forty-five minutes to make. My ranch dip recipe, which is used for the sauce, can be found on page 159.

Your bacon and beef pizza will be done when the cheese is melted, but if you want it to look and taste like a professional chef made it, place it under a broiler on high heat for three to five minutes to get the cheese to brown a bit on top. The broiled cheese looks super legit and adds flavor by caramelizing the sugars in the cheese.

This recipe is best served fresh, but it can be stored in the fridge for a few days and is best reheated in the oven or an air fryer.

Your imagination and preferences will guide you regarding variations or substitutions for this recipe. If you desire, you can use a traditional marinara sauce or even a hollandaise sauce (found on page 165) instead of the ranch. When it comes to the cheese, feel free to experiment. You could use ricotta for a gourmet-style pizza or a provolone/ mozzarella mix. It's up to you to discover what you like.

I love how you can mix and match different types of pizza toppings. Try adding caramelized onions or sautéed mushrooms or incorporating fresh herbs like basil or cilantro.

Difficulty Level: 2 out of 5 Meatballs

Prep Time: 5 Minutes

Cook Time: 10 Minutes

Servings: 1

Nutritional Facts: (Per Serving)
Calories 259
Protein 16g
Fat 20g
Total Carbohydrates

1 tablespoon of ranch dip

3 ounces of ground beef, cooked

1 ounce of bacon, extra crispy and crumbled

2 ounces of mozzarella cheese, shredded

Preheat oven to 400°F.

If your chicken-based pizza crust is cold, place it on the center rack of your oven and bake for 5 minutes at 400°F.

Spread the ranch dip evenly on the pizza crust, then evenly distribute the ground beef.

Cover with the mozzarella and top with the bacon crumbles.

Bake for 6-10 minutes at 400°F or until the cheese is melted.

Remove from the oven, let cool for 3-5 minutes, then enjoy!

Chicken-Based Pizza Crust

With forty-three grams of protein and only one carbohydrate, this chicken-based pizza crust recipe is perfect for anyone following a ketogenic or carnivore diet. The best part is that it tastes good and is good for you.

You can use freshly cooked chicken for this recipe, but I recommend canned chicken because it's easier. If you use canned chicken breast, you'll want to ensure you get as much of the liquid out as possible. Open the can, and with the lid still in place, flip the can over and squeeze the lid against the chicken to press out the liquid.

Use your hands or a fork to shred the chicken and spread it on the parchment paper so it can dry properly.

When you form the crust, press down on the chicken mixture to form one even solid mass. Ensure the edges are fully incorporated into the rest of the crust so it doesn't fall apart when you eat it.

When the crust is done baking, it should look dry. If it is still moist, flip it over and continue baking until it dries out. This step will help form a solid base for your pizza.

This pizza crust can be made ahead of time and stored in the fridge for up to one week. However, you must bake or air fry it before using it.

This recipe does not call for any seasoning, but you can include some if you like. I recommend garlic and onion powder, but you can add any spices you like, maybe some red pepper flakes if you want to kick it up a notch.

You can also use this pizza crust as you would crackers by cutting it into smaller pieces. You may need to bake it longer as well. You can eat your chicken crackers with egg or chicken salad.

Difficulty Level: 2 out of 5 Meatballs

Prep Time: 5 Minutes

Cook Time: 20 Minutes

Servings: 2

Nutritional Facts: (Per Serving)
Calories 349
Protein 43g
Fat 17g
Total Carbohydrates

7-10 ounces of canned chicken

1 ounce of parmesan cheese, shredded

1 egg

Preheat the oven to 350°F.

Drain the canned chicken, getting as much moisture out as possible.

Break up and spread the chicken on a parchment paper-lined baking sheet and bake at 350°F for 10 minutes.

Remove from the oven and place in a mixing bowl. Increase the heat of the oven to 400°F.

Add the parmesan cheese and egg to the bowl with the chicken and mix until well combined.

Dump the mixture onto a parchment-paper-lined baking sheet and spread it out to form a 5-inch by 10-inch rectangle. Press down on the mixture to form a 1/2-inch thick crust.

Bake for 8-10 minutes at 400°F.

If the crust is still moist, flip it over and bake for another 3-5 minutes.

Let the crust cool on a baking rack and cut in half lengthwise to form 2 personal pizza crusts.

Guilt-Free Grilled Teriyaki Chicken

I have adapted this recipe from traditional teriyaki chicken to make it healthier without sacrificing flavor. I have done this by removing the added sugar and the soy sauce and replacing them both with coconut aminos. I love cooking with coconut aminos because they are soy-free and add a note of sweetness. It is a liquid made with the fermented sap of the coconut palm and sea salt.

If you don't have a grill or the weather is not conducive to outdoor cooking, you can bake your chicken in the oven and then broil it at the end to get that beautiful char, or you can make them in a pan over the stove, but the clean up can be a pain, that's why I prefer the grill.

The longer you marinate the chicken, the more flavorful it will be. You can use the marinade to baste the thighs while cooking, but remember it was exposed to raw chicken, and to avoid getting food poisoning, you need to stop basting about halfway through the cooking process to allow the heat to kill off the harmful bacteria.

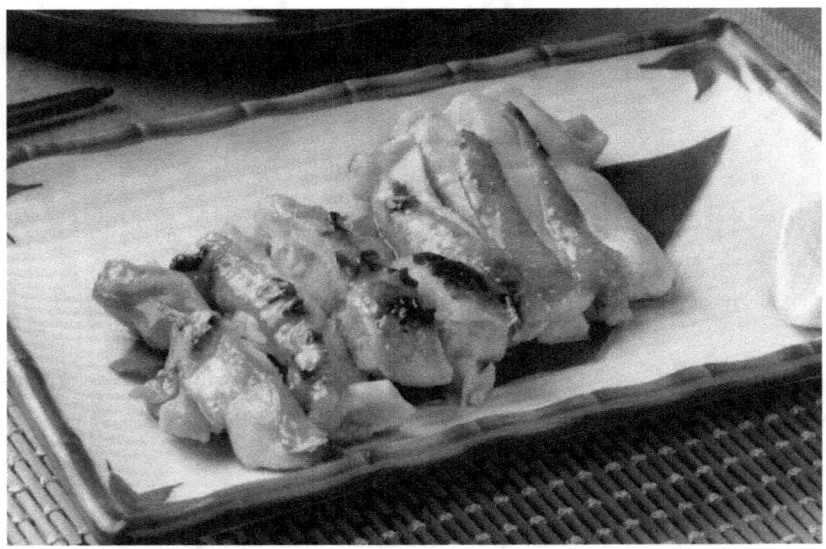

You can store your teriyaki chicken in the fridge for up to a week or freeze it for up to three months. You can use this recipe for meal prep by freezing individual portions. When ready to use them, pull out what you need. They will also defrost faster in smaller portions, especially if you flatten them out before freezing.

As always, I encourage you to make this recipe your own by modifying it to fit your tastes. Add some sriracha sauce or a few slices of Thai chili to the marinade if you want it spicy. If you don't like ginger, skip it. This is your show, so make it how you like it!

Get good grill marks by getting your grill nice and hot before cooking. The char will add an additional layer of flavor and a bit of crunch if you do it right.

This dish is excellent on its own, but it also can be served on a salad, on top of steamed rice, or as an ingredient in fried rice.

Difficulty Level: 2 out of 5 Meatballs

Prep Time: 5 Minutes

Cook Time: 10 Minutes

Servings: 3

Nutritional Facts:
(Per Serving)

Calories 451

Protein 58g

Fat 17g

Total Carbohydrates 10g

2 cloves of garlic, minced

1 inch of ginger root, minced

1 tablespoon of sesame oil

1/2 cup of coconut aminos

1 tablespoon of rice vinegar

1 tablespoon of Worcestershire sauce

1/4 teaspoon of pepper

2 pounds of chicken thighs

1 tablespoon of toasted sesame seeds

1 tablespoon of chives, finely sliced

Combine the garlic, ginger, sesame oil, coconut aminos, rice vinegar, Worcestershire sauce, and pepper in a large container or zip-top bag.

Stir to mix the marinade, then add chicken thighs. Seal and let marinate in the fridge for at least one hour or overnight.

Preheat your grill on high heat.

Grill chicken thighs for approximately 5 minutes on each side or until an internal temperature of 165 ° is reached and the outside of the chicken has started to char.

Garnish with toasted sesame seeds and chives.

Traditional Barbacoa: A Taste of Mexico

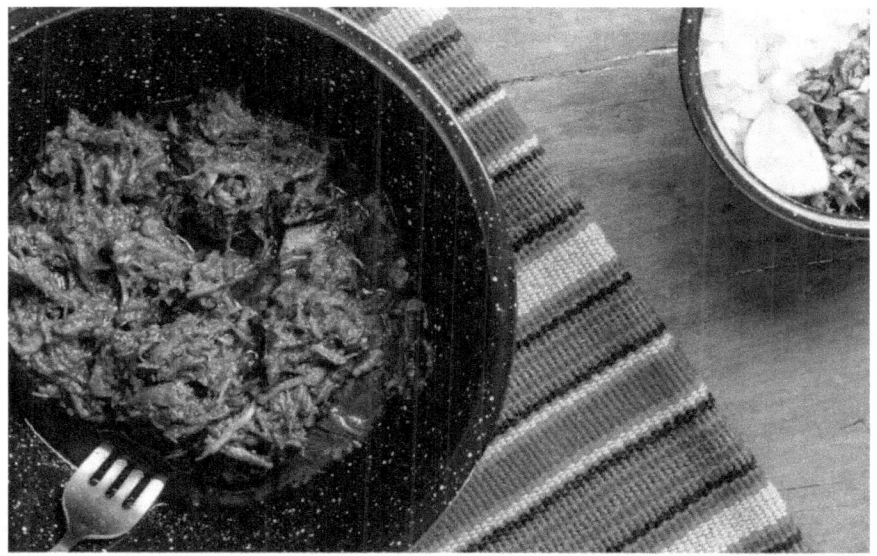

Barbacoa has deep roots in Caribbean and Mexican culinary traditions, and its origins trace back to the indigenous Taíno people of the Caribbean. The term "barbacoa" comes from the Taíno word "barabicu" which means meat cooked on a wooden structure over an open fire. This is also where the word barbeque comes from. This cooking method spread and evolved throughout Mexico and Central America.

In Mexico, barbacoa is often associated with celebrations and special occasions like quenceneras or weddings. Different regions have their own variations, too. In central Mexico, it's common to use sheep or goat, and in the northern regions, beef is more commonly used. In the Yucatan, a similar dish called "cochinita pibil" uses pork marinated in achiote and sour orange wrapped in banana leaves and cooked in a pit.

Traditionally, Mexican barbacoa involves slow-cooking meat, usually beef, lamb, or goat, in a pit covered with agave leaves. This method allows the meat to become tender and absorb the flavors from the leaves and the earth. The process is time-consuming, often taking several hours, resultinmg in flavorful, juicy meat.

I have taken this traditional, time-consuming dish and made it relatively fast and easy to prepare while preserving the authentic flavor using a pressure cooker. You can also use a slow cooker or a pit if you like, but I argue it's just as good when made my way.

If you live anywhere in Southern California, the chili peppers used in this dish can be found at almost any grocery store in the ethnic food aisle. If you live somewhere without a strong Hispanic influence, you may need to order your chili peppers online. They come dried, so they are lightweight and will last a long time in your pantry.

You can remove the seeds from the chili peppers if you want it less spicy or substitute the arbol chili for chili de California (seeds removed) for an even less spicy option.

You can also substitute the chuck roast for beef stew meat for this recipe, but you must reduce the cooking time.

This dish will last in the fridge for up to a week or in a freezer for up to three months. If you freeze it, hold off on frying it in the beef tallow until you are ready to eat it.

Barbacoa goes excellent in tacos, with Mexican rice (A tomato and chicken bullion flavored rice fried in oil before cooking), or on its own with diced onion and cilantro.

Difficulty Level: 3 out of 5 Meatballs

Prep Time: 30 Minutes

Cook Time: 1.5 Hours

Servings: 6

Nutritional Facts: (Per Serving)
Calories 730
Protein 75g
Total Fat 45g
Total Carbohydrates

3-5 pounds of chuck roast

1/2 cup of beef broth

4 tablespoons of beef tallow

2 guajillo peppers, dried

1 arbol pepper, dried

1/2 teaspoon of cumin

1 teaspoon of oregano

1/2 onion, diced

1 bulb of garlic, minced

2 teaspoons of salt

6 whole black peppercorns

3 bay leaves

1 tablespoon of Worcestershire sauce

Place the beef tallow in a saucepan over medium heat. Add the onion once the tallow has melted and cook for 1 minute. Add the garlic and let cook another minute. Stir the garlic and onion, then add the chili peppers; take care not to burn the peppers as they toast quickly.

Place all ingredients, except the chuck roast, into a blender and blend until smooth to create the marinade. Let cool for at least 1 hour. Then, place the chuck roast into a zip-top bag or other container along with the marinade. Seal and let it marinate overnight in the refrigerator.

Place the chuck roast and marinade in a pressure cooker, cook on high pressure for 45 minutes, then carefully release the pressure.

Remove meat from the pot and continue cooking the juices on soup/stew mode for 30 minutes to 1 hour or until reduced by half.

Once the chuck roast has cooled, shred it by hand or with two forks.

Before serving, heat 1 tablespoon of tallow in a skillet over high heat and pan-fry the shredded beef. Do this in smaller batches to get a crispy crust on the beef.

Place a portion of the shredded beef into a bowl, add some of the sauce, and serve with diced onions and cilantro, and enjoy!

DAIRY

When we talk about protein-rich foods, dairy doesn't always get the spotlight, but it can add variety to a low-carb diet. In this chapter, I've included a few standout recipes where dairy takes center stage. But you'll also find milk and cheeses playing supporting roles in many other dishes throughout this cookbook. I always recommend opting for whole raw milk and aged cheeses whenever you can get your hands on them.

Why whole milk? The fat content in whole raw milk is more than just delicious—it's a powerful, sustainable energy source. It fuels your body for longer periods, which can be a game changer if you're looking to stay full and satisfied between meals. Plus, this kind of fat supports hormone production and keeps your brain sharp. You won't get these benefits from low-fat milk or heavily processed milk alternatives.

Why raw milk? The beneficial enzymes, along with the vitamins and minerals in raw milk, help our bodies break it down and absorb its nutrients. Sadly, these enzymes get destroyed during pasteurization, stripping the milk of much of its natural benefits. For those who tolerate dairy well, whole raw milk and cheeses can be an incredibly nourishing part of a balanced diet.

If raw milk isn't available to you, don't worry. High-quality organic dairy is still a good option, especially when it's full fat. In the end, the goal is to use whole, nutrient-dense ingredients. So whether it's a simple drizzle of cream in your morning coffee or a tangy aged cheese in a hearty casserole, don't overlook the power that dairy can bring to the table.

Blender Ice Cream

Like many of us, I loved eating ice cream while growing up. It was always a special treat to go to the local ice cream shop, try a few flavors, and get a few scoops of my favorites. Unfortunately, most ice creams contain a ton of added sugar and artificial flavors. Luckily, this ice cream recipe has no added sugar, is all-natural, and can be made with only a common kitchen blender.

I use a Vitamix blender to make this recipe, but you can use any blender or food processor. I've made this recipe in a small smoothie-style blender like a magic bullet. You will have to make this recipe in two separate batches if you use a smaller blender like this, and you may have to pick up the blender and shake it up and down to get the mixture to combine correctly. It will taste just as good but takes a little more work.

The key to this recipe is to continually scrape down the sides of the blender pitcher to incorporate any bits that get stuck there. Once you add the cream, you must blend the mixture on the slowest setting to avoid the mixture from accumulating on the sides of the pitcher. Once the mixture starts to come together, you can try ramping up the blender's speed in tiny increments to speed up the process, but if you go too fast, the mixture will get stuck to the sides of the blender pitcher.

After you blend the berries, they should have a pulp-like consistency. Blending the berries first helps ensure a smooth texture in the end product. If you use a smaller blender, it can be helpful to chop the berries into quarter-inch pieces by hand before blending them.

This recipe does not store well. If you leave it in the freezer for more than an hour, it will become rock-hard and lose its creamy texture. You can still eat it by scraping the surface with a spoon, but it will be more like shaved ice.

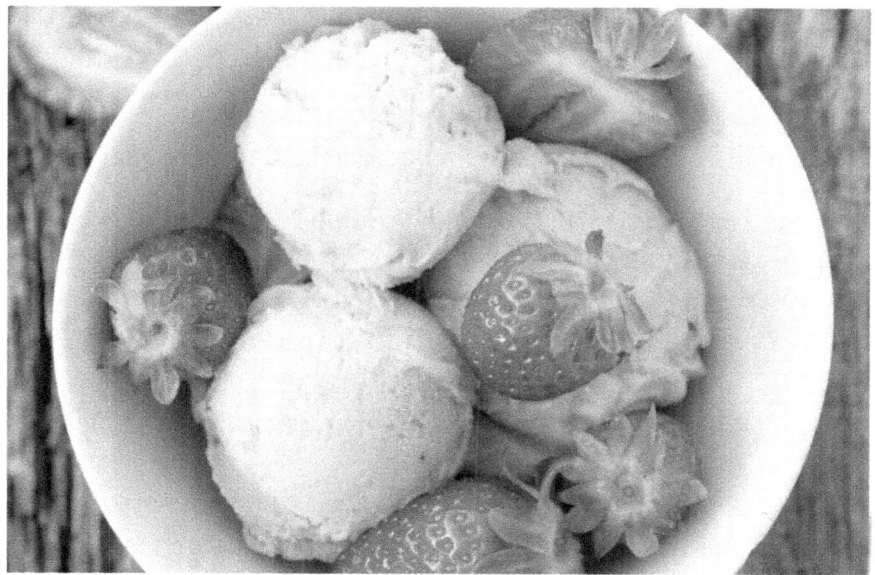

I recommend making this dish while you prepare your dinner so that it will be ready by the time you're done with dinner and ready for a sweet treat. If you don't have time or can't wait, you can still enjoy your blender ice cream without the additional time in the freezer. A tip for this would be to get the cream as cold as possible before blending your ice cream.

There are many ways to customize this recipe. You can use any fruit you like. You can use fresh fruit, but you must dice it into one-inch pieces, spread them out on a parchment-lined baking sheet, and place them in the freezer for at least 2 hours or until the fruit is frozen solid.

Suggested flavors include:

- Raspberry

- Strawberry

- Banana and strawberry

- Mango

- Banana with chocolate protein powder

If you are sensitive to dairy, you can substitute the heavy cream with coconut cream. This variation is very tasty; however, the coconut cream does not whip up as much as the heavy cream and the end product will have a slightly different texture and taste like coconut.

You can replace the fruit with ice cubes made from a protein shake if you do not eat plant materials. To do this, mix your protein powder of choice with whole milk and freeze it in an ice cube tray. When making your ice cream, substitute the frozen fruit with the protein ice cubes. This variation is best suited for a commercial-grade blender like a Vitamix.

Need more protein? Add a few egg yolks or half a scoop of protein powder to the cream before blending. Traditional ice cream recipes call for egg yolks, so if you use them, you will have a more decadent and creamy end product, similar to traditional ice cream, plus the additional protein.

Difficulty Level: 1 out of 5 Meatballs

Prep Time: 10 Minutes

Cook Time: None

Servings: 2

Nutritional Facts:
(Per Serving)
Calories 255
Protein 2g
Fat 20g
Total Carbohydrates 17g

5 ounces of frozen blueberries

5 ounces of frozen strawberries

⅔ cup (4 ounces) of heavy cream

Chill 2 small serving bowls in the freezer.

Add the frozen strawberries and blueberries to the blender pitcher. Blend at medium speed until no big chunks are left, about 30 seconds.

Add the heavy cream into the blender pitcher, use a rubber spatula to scrape down the sides, and incorporate the berries at the bottom with the cream.

Blend on low for 1 minute. Scrape down the sides and bottom of the pitcher with the rubber spatula again and blend the mixture until all ingredients are well incorporated. This should take 1-2 minutes.

Repeat the previous step as needed to achieve a smooth and uniform texture.

Transfer your ice cream to the pre-chilled bowls and place them in the freezer for 1 hour.

After 1 hour, take the ice cream out of the freezer and scrape the sides and bottoms of each bowl to incorporate the outer frozen layer using a spoon, and enjoy!

Parmesan and Cottage Cheese Chips

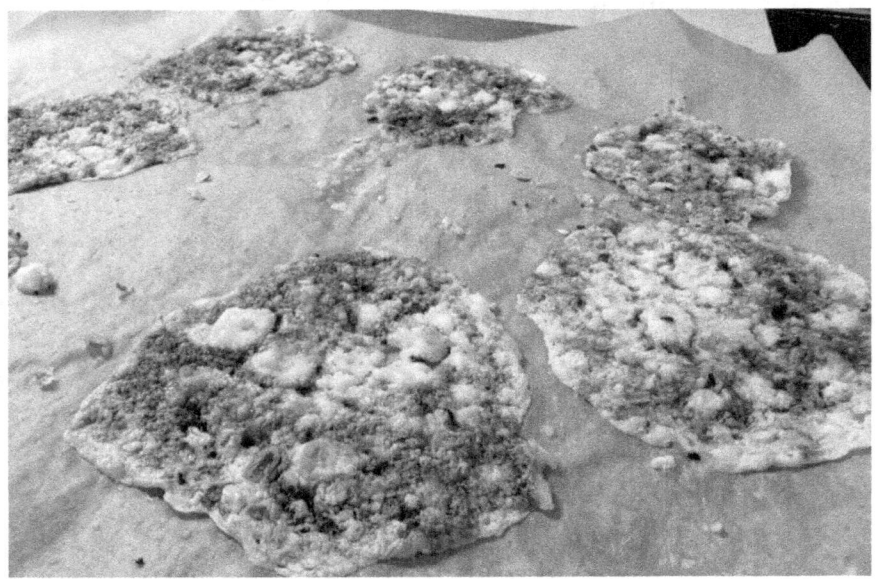

These parmesan and cottage cheese chips are super low-carb and are a fantastic dip delivery system. You can even make miniature hard-shell tacos with them!

Cottage cheese chips have been all the rage online recently, and that is where I discovered this recipe. However, I have modified the original recipe by adding parmesan cheese to give the chips more rigidity, and I make them in the microwave for convenience. The original recipe calls to bake the chips in the oven for forty minutes, then rotate the pan and bake for another forty minutes. Who has the time to make only nine chips every hour and a half? That's ridiculous. With this recipe, you can make eight chips in under ten minutes.

The only equipment needed to make this recipe is a microwave and parchment paper.

When placing the dollops of cottage cheese on the parchment paper, use your finger or another spoon to help remove the cottage cheese from the measuring spoon.

You will know the chips are done when they are dry and have started to turn light brown. If you want to use the chips as mini hard-shell tacos, fold them over or put them in a taco shell holder before they cool. These chips are best eaten fresh and will become soggy if stored in an air-tight container.

Parmesan and cottage cheese chips are delicious on their own, but they are even better with the everything bagel seasoning. You can customize these chips with your seasoning of choice, but beware, cottage cheese is salty on its own, so if you choose to use another type of seasoning, use one with less salt. You can also add cheddar or other cheeses if you like.

Each microwave is different, so you may have to experiment with cooking times. Start with three minutes and then check them for doneness. If they are not done, continue cooking in one-minute intervals and check for doneness between them.

These chips are very tasty alone but can also be used as a dip delivery system. I enjoy them with my creamy buffalo chicken featured in the creamy buffalo chicken wrap recipe on page 95.

Difficulty Level: 1 out of 5 Meatballs

Prep Time: 1 Minute

Cook Time: 3-5 Minutes

Servings: 1

Nutritional Facts:
(Per Serving)

Calories 298

Protein 29g

Fat 17g

Total Carbohydrates

1/2 cup of cottage cheese

1/2 cup of shredded parmesan cheese

1 tablespoon of everything bagel seasoning

Place a cutting board on the counter. Cut a piece of parchment paper that will fit flat in your microwave and place it on the cutting board.

Place 1 tablespoon dollops of cottage cheese 2 inches apart on the parchment paper. You should be able to make approximately 8 chips.

Flatten each dollop of cottage cheese to the size of a half dollar using the back of a spoon to form the chips. Sprinkle 1 tablespoon of parmesan cheese on top of each chip, then sprinkle some everything bagel seasoning on top of the cheese.

Using the cutting board to support the parchment paper, transfer the parchment paper into the microwave and microwave for 3 minutes.

Check the chips for doneness. You will know when they are done when the chips are dry and have started to brown.

If they are not done, microwave one minute at a time until the desired doneness is achieved.

Remove from the microwave, let cool for 3 minutes and enjoy!

Creamy Strawberry Delight

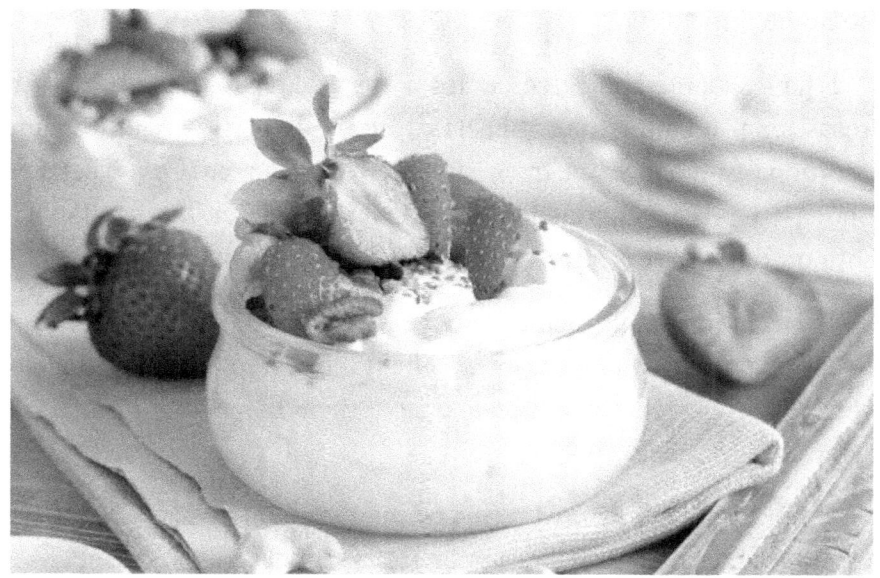

This recipe is a perfect blend of flavors with the creamy tartness of the Greek yogurt and the natural sweetness of strawberries. The addition of vanilla protein powder adds flavor and boosts the protein content of the Greek yogurt further, ensuring you stay full and satisfied with this scrumptious treat.

The strawberries add a burst of flavor and are packed with antioxidants, vitamins, and fiber, promoting overall health. Whether you enjoy this dish as a post-workout snack or a guilt-free dessert after dinner, it's sure to become a favorite. Try adding a pinch of cinnamon as a flavor enhancer.

This recipe calls for either fresh or frozen strawberries. I recommend frozen because when you freeze them, you rupture the cell walls of the strawberries, releasing additional flavor.

This recipe is a bit higher in carbohydrates than most of the others in this cookbook, so if you are eating a low-carb diet, be mindful that each serving contains twenty-four grams of carbs.

I recommend using an animal-based protein powder like whey or casein, we are just not optimized to utilize plant proteins. I also would like to say that protein powder is a processed food, and consumption should be limited.

I have adapted this recipe from the beloved Mexican dessert Fresas con crema witch translates to strawberries with cream. Traditionally made from fresh strawberries, sour cream, sweetened condensed milk, evaporated milk, and vanilla extract. My version has more protein and less sugar making it a healthier option.

You can make this dish ahead of time as it will store in the fridge for about a week or so. This an excellent meal prep recipe as you can prepare a few batches at a time and store them in small mason jars as a grab and go snack.

If you don't like strawberries or they are out of season you can substitute them for other berries or fruits. Blueberries or raspberries would be a good substitutes. You could even skip the fruit or berries all together and replace the vanilla protein powder with a chocolate protein powder for a chocolate pudding like experience.

Difficulty Level: 1 out of 5 Meatballs

Prep Time: 5 Minutes

Cook Time: None

Servings: 1

Nutritional Facts: (Per Serving)
Calories 283
Protein 40g
Fat 3g
Total Carbohydrates 24g

1 cup of Greek yogurt

1 scoop of vanilla protein powder

1 cup strawberries (fresh or frozen), sliced

In a medium bowl, combine the Greek yogurt and protein powder. Stir until the protein powder is fully incorporated.

Gently fold the sliced strawberries into the yogurt mixture.

Enjoy immediately, or chill in the refrigerator for a refreshing snack.

EGGS

E ggs are a personal favorite of mine because they're incredibly versatile and can be prepared in so many ways. Whether scrambled, poached, boiled, baked, or fried, eggs can fit seamlessly into almost every meal. Eggs also play a vital role—binding ingredients and adding structure to other recipes. But there's more to eggs than just culinary magic; they're nutritional powerhouses too.

When it comes to eggs, I always recommend using whole eggs—not just the whites. The yolk is where the magic is; it's packed with healthy fats, including cholesterol, which plays a crucial role in hormone production and supports brain and nervous system health. Cutting out yolks means missing out on these essential benefits.

Eggs are also loaded with key vitamins and minerals, like vitamin B12, choline, and selenium, which contribute to energy production, liver function, and immune health. They also deliver a good balance of protein and fat, keeping you satisfied and fueled throughout your day.

In this chapter, you'll discover a variety of egg-based recipes, ranging from simple breakfast staples to more elaborate dishes. Whether making a quick omelet, egg bites, or sneaking an egg yolk into your ice cream, eggs are a cornerstone of the Protein Lifestyle.

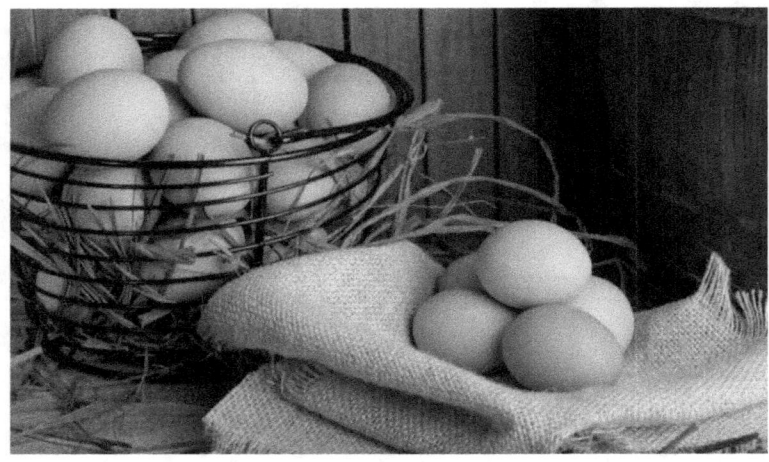

Bacon and Cheddar Egg Bites

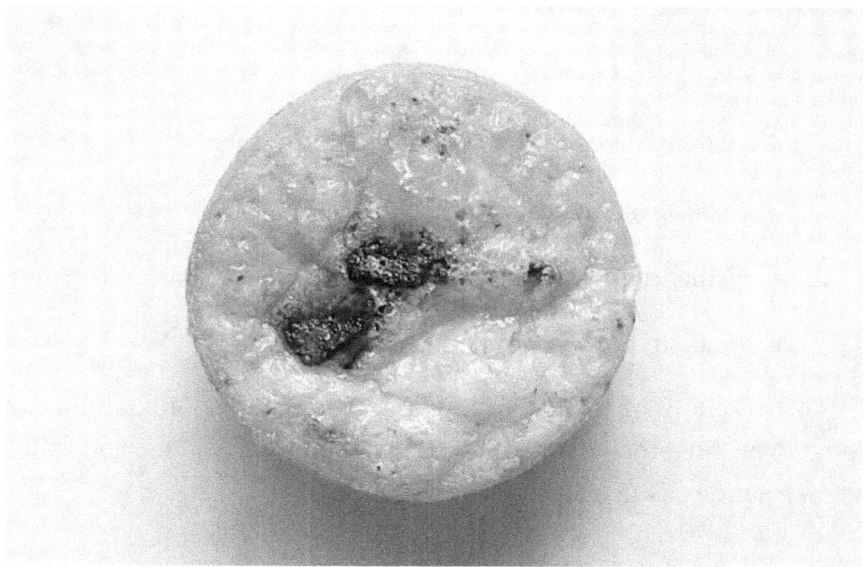

Egg bites are a convenient and portable dish you can eat as a snack or a meal in themselves. This recipe packs a whopping forty-six grams of protein and only five grams of carbohydrates per serving.

A muffin tin or silicone muffin liners are used to form the egg bites. I prefer the silicone muffin liners because they are easier to clean, and you can leave the egg bites in them until you're ready to eat them. A traditional muffin tin will work well just make sure you grease it with butter before baking.

When checking for doneness, stick a toothpick into one of the egg bites, and if it comes out clean, it is done, like you would when baking a cake. If not, continue to bake them and recheck for doneness often to avoid overcooking them.

Egg bites are excellent for meal prepping and can be stored in the fridge for up to one week, and are easily reheated in the microwave.

Their are so many options when it comes to customizing your egg bites. You can replace the bacon with any meat you like; the same goes for the cheese. You can also add vegetables if your into that sort of thing.

Variation suggestions:

- Pesto and tomato

- Caramelized onion and breakfast sausage

- Sun-dried tomato and basil

- Mushroom and spinach

- Bacon, cream cheese, jalapeno

To make any of these variations, replace the bacon and cheddar from the original recipe with the your ingredients of choice and follow the instructions as usual.

Difficulty Level: 2 out of 5 Meatballs

Prep Time: 5 Minutes

Cook Time: 20 Minutes

Servings: 3

Nutritional Facts:
(Per Serving)
Calories 772
Protein 46g
Fat 61g
Total Carbohydrates

12 eggs

3/4 cup cottage cheese

1/2 a pound of bacon, cooked and crumbled

1 cup cheddar cheese, shredded

1 teaspoon of salt

1/2 teaspoon of pepper

Preheat oven to 350°F.

Place all ingredients in a medium-sized bowl and mix until well combined.

Grease 6 muffin tin wells with butter or use 6 silicone muffin liners; fill each well 3/4 full with the egg mixture.

Bake at 350°F for 15 to 20 minutes or until a toothpick comes out clean.

Let cool for 5 minutes and enjoy!

Hard Poached Egg Salad

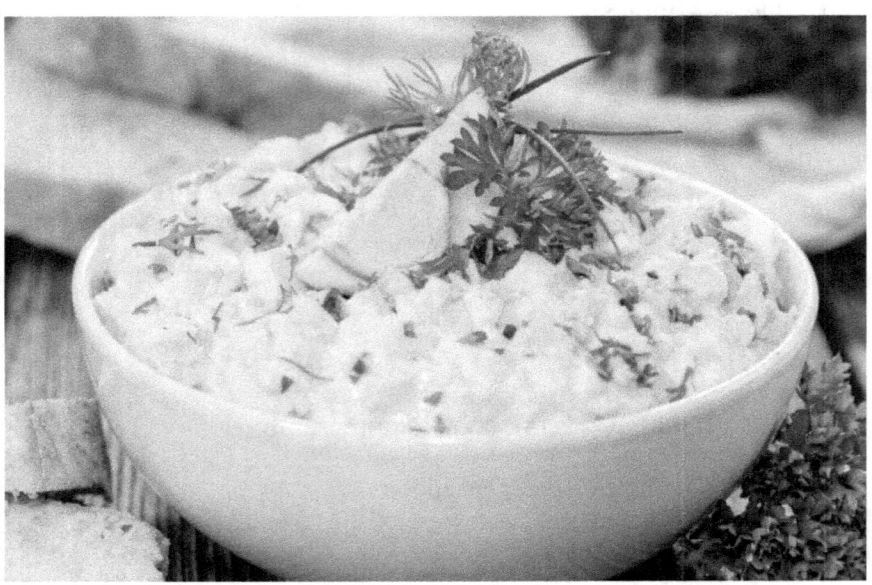

This recipe utilizes hard-poached eggs instead of hard-boiled eggs and includes cottage cheese for added texture and some additional protein. You can still use hard boiled if you like, but I don't have the time or patience to peel them, so I use this method.

What are hard-poached eggs?

I'm glad you asked. They are eggs cooked in simmering water with a bit of vinegar in it and cooked until the yolk is hard. See page 138 for my perfectly poached egg recipe, but cook them longer to get firm yolks.

A bean masher will help to mash up the eggs but this can also be accomplished with a fork.

This hard-poached egg salad will last three to five days in the fridge.

For extra flavor and a little kick try adding some garlic chili sauce or chili onion crunch. If you want to take this recipe to another level try adding some fresh chives or dill.

Difficulty Level: 2 out of 5 Meatballs

Prep Time: 5 Minutes

Cook Time: None

Servings: 1

Nutritional Facts:
(Per Serving)

Calories 1041

Protein 57g

Fat 83g

Total Carbohydrates 10g

8 eggs, hard poached

1/4 cup of cottage cheese

1/4 cup of mayonnaise

2 tablespoons of stone ground mustard

1 teaspoon of smoked paprika

1 tablespoon Worcestershire sauce

1 tablespoon everything bagel seasoning

Place the hard poached eggs in a large bowl and mash with a fork.

Add the rest of the ingredients and mix everything together until it is uniform in consistency.

Enjoy alone or in a cottage cheese flatbread wrap, found on page 97.

Perfectly Poached Eggs

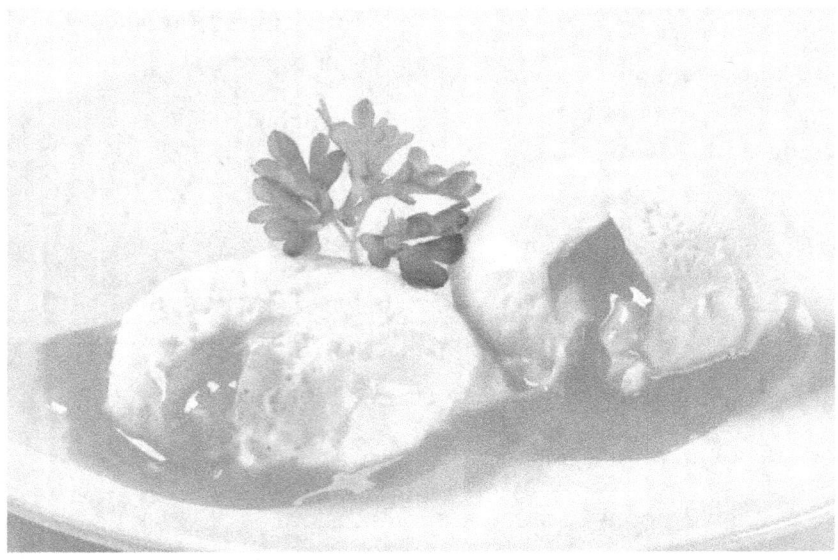

Making perfectly poached eggs is a simple and an elegant way to step up your game in the kitchen. Traditionally served with breakfast dishes like eggs Benedict or my Turkey Croquettes Benedict (Found on page 161), poached eggs can be a great addition to any meal.

Stemming from French cuisine, the term "poached" originated from the French word "poché," which can be translated to English as "pocket" or "small pouch." This method of cooking eggs in simmering water produces a delicate yet decadent dish that produces a firm white with a runny golden yolk. Don't fret if you're squeamish about the thought of runny yolks. You can poach your eggs for longer if you prefer a firmer yolk.

Traditionally, poached eggs are made in a saucepan over the stove, but you can also make them in a microwave. Either way, you will need a slotted spoon to remove the poached eggs from the water.

The key to creating a perfectly poached egg is to create a vortex in the water inside your pot. Do this by swirling the simmering water in the pot with a spoon and immediately adding the egg. This will give you an excellent uniform shape in your end product. The egg will stay together better, and you will avoid those wispy strands of egg whites.

Gently crack your egg into a small bowl, ensuring not to break the yolk. This can be achieved by tapping the shell against a hard surface just above or below the egg's equator and gently place in a small bowl. When placing the egg into the water, get the edge of the bowl as close to the water as possible. If some of the water goes into the bowl, it's all good. Doing this slowly and carefully is critical.

If you make more than one egg at a time, you can skip the vortex method and use a spoon to help gather the whites in one mass. Add your eggs in a clockwise direction to help you keep track of the order in which you place them in the water. This is the order in which you will remove the eggs, so the timing is right for each. Do not add more than four eggs per batch; the water will drop below a simmer, and your eggs will not cook properly.

Adding a bit of vinegar to the water raises the acidity, which helps keep the whites together by forming a thin layer around the egg. You can make poached eggs without vinegar, but it will help with getting that perfectly poached egg.

You can make poached eggs ahead of time by only cooking them for three minutes and then placing them in an ice water bath. They can be stored in the fridge in the water for about three to four days. To reheat them, place them in boiling water for thirty seconds each.

Serve your poached eggs with salt and pepper on top of a slice of sourdough toast, as part of a Lyonnaise salad, or on top of a juicy steak.

Difficulty Level: 2 out of 5 Meatballs

Prep Time: 1 Minute

Cook Time: 3 Minutes

Servings: 1

Nutritional Facts:
(Per Serving)

Calories 72

Protein 6g

Fat 4g

Total Carbohydrates

1 egg

1 tablespoon of white vinegar

Filtered water

Pour the white vinegar into a saucepan, add 3 to 4 inches of water, then place on the stovetop over medium heat.

Carefully crack the egg into a small bowl.

Once the water has reached a soft boil (190°F), use a spoon to stir the water, creating a vortex.

Gently place the egg into the swirling water and let poach for 3 minutes.

Remove the egg with a slotted spoon and place it on a paper towel to soak up the residual water, then serve immediately or place in ice water for later use.

LAMB

While I've only included one lamb recipe in this cookbook, lamb is a fantastic protein option that deserves a place in any well-rounded diet. Sheep, like beef, are ruminant animals with multiple stomachs. This unique digestive system helps ruminants naturally filter out any toxins that may be present in their diet, resulting in cleaner meat.

If you're new to cooking with lamb, you'll likely come across lamb from the Netherlands, which is an excellent choice. Dutch lamb is often raised holistically, fed on grass, and kept free from antibiotics and hormones, factors that align perfectly with the Protein Lifestyle's focus on quality, nutrient-dense food.

Lamb is known for its rich, savory flavor and is leaner than beef. This means paying attention when cooking is essential, overcooking can dry it out quickly. When done right, lamb can elevate your meals, adding a depth of flavor that's hard to beat.

While this chapter offers just a taste of what lamb can bring to the table, I encourage you to explore beyond the recipe I've provided. Try experimenting with a rack of lamb for a show-stopping dinner or grill up some lamb loin chops for a quick, flavorful meal. With its distinct taste and nutrient profile, lamb is a great addition to your diet and a delicious way to diversify your protein sources.

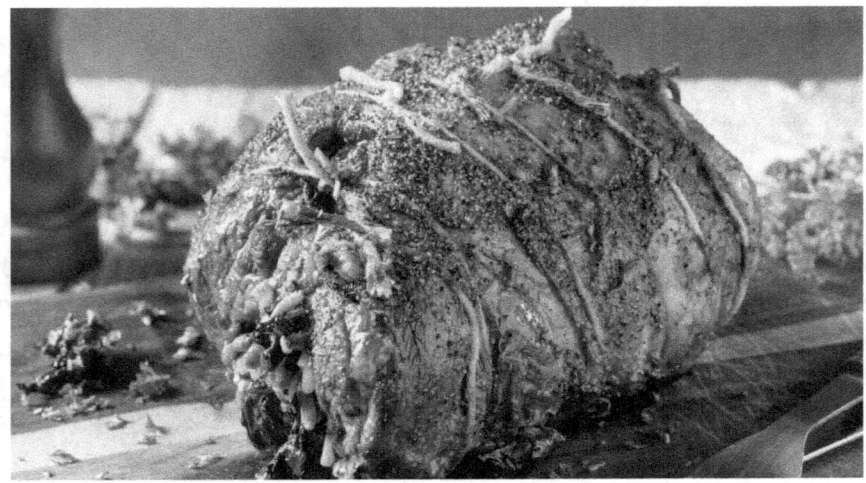

Roasted Leg of Lamb with Rosemary and Garlic

A roasted leg of lamb sounds intimidating, but it is one of the easier recipes in this cookbook, and it will truly impress anyone you prepare it for. When you serve this roasted leg of lamb with a slice or two of seared queso fresco, it makes for an incredible low-carb meal

I highly recommend using a leave-in probe thermometer to monitor the temperature of the roast. These thermometers have a temperature alarm that will go off when a preset temperature is reached, allowing you to get a perfectly cooked leg of lamb with minimal effort. The key to success is to set the temperature alarm to one hundred and thirty degrees Fahrenheit. As soon as the alarm sounds, pull it from the oven, cover the roast with foil, and let it rest for fifteen minutes to allow the juices to redistribute within the meat. Since lamb is leaner, you'll want to preserve as much juice as possible. Once you pull the roast from the oven, the residual heat will continue to raise the temperature. This is why we set the alarm below the desired final cooking temperature.

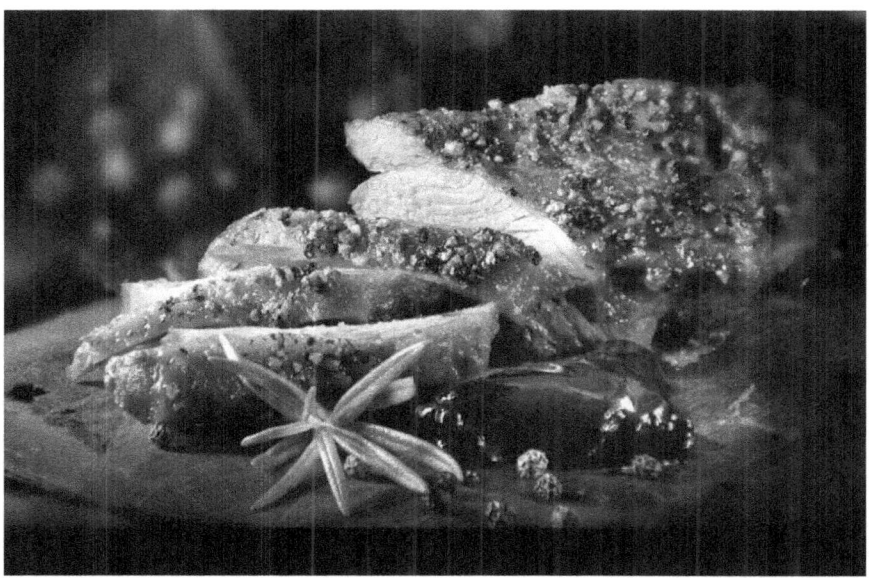

This lamb roast can be stored for about a week in the fridge, and I do not recommend freezing it due to its leanness. It will be tricky to reheat without drying it out. You can, however, freeze the uncooked lamb for future preparation without any issues

Feel free to use a bone-in leg of lamb for this recipe; it will add flavor, but you will need to roast it longer. This is a simple recipe, and if you want to add a few more levels of flavor, try making a wet rub by adding a tablespoon of Dijon mustard and a tablespoon of chopped fresh thyme leaves in addition to the garlic, rosemary, and olive oil.

I get bored of eating food like this without a side dish, and when you eat low-carb, keto, or carnivore, it can be hard to find sides that work. As I mentioned, I like to eat lamb with seared queso fresco. It's very easy to make. All you need to do is slice the cheese into one-inch-thick slices and throw it in a hot cast iron skillet with some clarified butter for about one minute per side or until it gets browned on each side. The key is to do this at the last minute because this cheese cools quickly, and once it does, it gets rubbery. You could also use any other grilling cheese like paneer, but I like queso fresco because it is cost-effective and can also be eaten fresh with many dishes.

Difficulty Level: 2 out of 5 Meatballs

Prep Time: 10 Minutes

Cook Time: 1 Hour

Servings: 5

Nutritional Facts:
(Per Serving)

Calories 396

Protein 59g

Fat 15g

Total Carbohydrates

1 boneless leg of lamb roast

1 tablespoon of olive oil

4 cloves of garlic, minced

1 tablespoon of fresh rosemary

1 tablespoon of salt

2 teaspoons of pepper

Preheat oven to 350°F.

Pat dry the roast and season with salt and pepper.

Rub the olive oil all over the roast, then rub in the garlic and rosemary. Place your roast with the fat side up on a baking sheet lined with aluminum foil.

Place into the oven for 45 minutes to 1 hour or until it reaches an internal temperature of 130°F.

Remove from oven, cover, and let rest for 15 minutes.

Slice against the grain and serve immediately with a slice of seared queso fresco.

PORK

Pork is an incredibly versatile protein that offers a wide range of flavors, textures, and cooking methods. From juicy pork chops to slow-cooked pulled pork, this meat fits seamlessly into various dishes, making it an essential part of the Protein Lifestyle. Whether you're grilling, roasting, braising, or curing it, pork brings something special to the table every time.

One of pork's standout qualities is the diversity of cuts available. You'll find leaner options like tenderloin, perfect for quick meals, and fattier cuts like pork belly or shoulder, which become melt-in-your-mouth tender when cooked low and slow. This balance of lean and fatty cuts makes it easy to tailor pork dishes to your dietary preferences.

I always recommend seeking out high-quality pork, preferably pasture-raised and free from hormones or antibiotics. When pigs are raised with care and allowed to forage naturally, the result is meat with superior flavor and nutrition.

Like other animal fats, the fat in pork provides lasting energy and helps you feel satisfied after meals. Plus, pork is rich in essential nutrients like B vitamins, zinc, and selenium, all supporting immune function and metabolism.

In this chapter, you'll discover a few ways to prepare pork, but the possibilities extend far beyond these pages. Whether grilling up some smoky ribs, sautéing pork chops, or slow-cooking a savory roast, pork is an excellent protein option for anyone embracing a protein-forward lifestyle. Dive in, experiment, and enjoy all the delicious possibilities pork offers.

Browned Butter and Bacon Bark

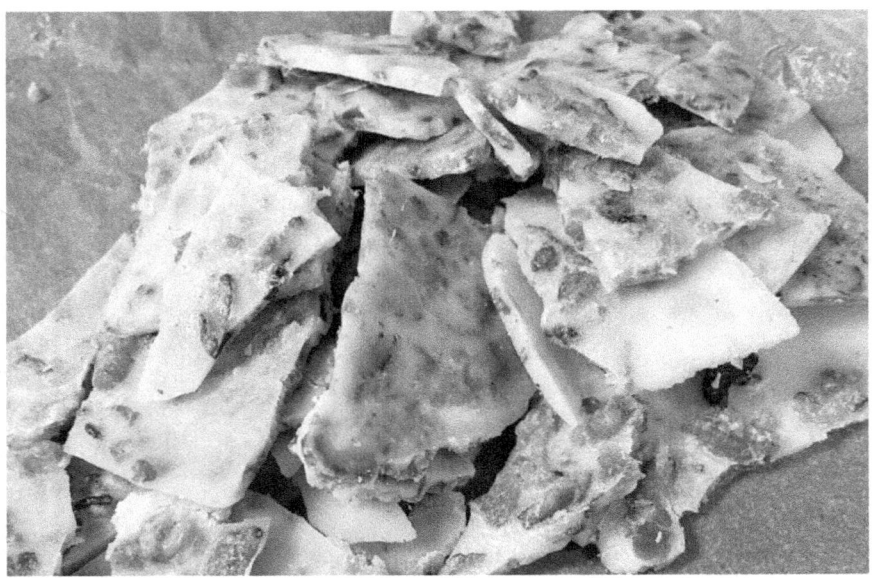

This recipe is an excellent choice for a sweet and savory treat. When you brown butter, its sugars caramelize, leaving you with a complex and rich flavor. When you match this with the savory flavor of bacon and top it off with coarse sea salt, you have a truly delightful combination.

This recipe is also known as carnivore crack or carnivore candy. It has its roots in the keto and carnivore communities as a high-fat and low-carb snack that fits perfectly into both the ketogenic and carnivore diets.

I like to use an air fryer to cook the bacon due to its speed and easy cleanup, but if you don't have one, don't fret. You can cook the bacon in a skillet, on a griddle, or in the oven on a baking sheet.

You will want to make sure to get your bacon as crispy as possible so it will hold up when you add the butter. There is a thin line between perfectly crispy and burnt bacon, so watch your bacon very closely towards the end of the cooking process to make sure you do not cross that line. Make your bacon beforehand to allow it to cool before browning the butter. My Bacon Twists is perfect for this and can be found immediately after this recipe.

Making browned butter is simple but can quickly burn, so you must pay close attention during the entire process. Using a light-colored pan like a stainless or white bottom skillet will help you monitor the color of the butter. Make sure to constantly stir and scrape the bottom of the pan so the butter heats evenly and the milk solids don't burn. Once your butter has browned, make sure to remove it from the pan immediately, as the residual heat from the pan can burn the butter. My browned butter recipe can be found on page 149. So, have your baking sheet with the bacon crumbles ready to go.

If you want to add more depth to this recipe try adding a handful of roughly chopped and toasted nuts like pecans or almonds. You can also try adding some vanilla extract and a dash of cinnamon for an added level of flavor.

You can store your bark in the refrigerator for up to one week or freeze it for three months.

This is a very rich dish and this recipe makes fourteen servings, each serving is approximately four inches by four inches across, therefore if you break your bark up into two inch pieces, a serving would be two pieces. Eat is slowly and savor the delicious flavor of each bite to get the full experience.

Difficulty Level: 3 out of 5 Meatballs

Prep Time: 5 Minutes

Cook Time: None

Servings: 14

Nutritional Facts:
(Per Serving)
Calories 217
Protein 3g
Total Fat 22g
Total Carbohydrates

1 pack of bacon, cooked, extra crispy

1 batch of browned butter

1 tablespoon of course sea salt

Crumble bacon into small pieces and spread it out evenly on a parchment paper-lined baking sheet.

Pour the browned butter over the bacon crumbles and sprinkle the salt evenly across the surface.

Put the backing sheet in the freezer for about 2 hours or until it has solidified.

Once the bark has hardened, cut it into 2-inch squares and enjoy.

Bacon Twists

1 12-16 ounce package of bacon

Preheat the air fryer to 400°F

Prepare the bacon by draping a piece of bacon over your index finger, grasping it with your other hand, and twisting your finger around so the bacon becomes twisted around itself. Continue this method with the rest of the bacon.

Place the bacon twists in the air fryer basket in one layer.

Air fry for 15-20 minutes, flipping the bacon halfway through cooking.

Continue cooking the bacon as needed until crispy.

Place the bacon on a baking sheet to cool for 5 minutes. Then enjoy the wonder of bacon, or use it in other recipes as directed!

Browned Butter

2 sticks of unsalted butter

Place a sauté pan over medium heat and add the butter.

Continually stir the butter for 5 to 10 minutes, or until the butter has turned a chestnut brown color and has a nutty aroma.

Use as a dip for crispy pork belly bites, on top of steaks, or in my Browned Butter and Bacon Bark recipe.

Authentic Al Pastor

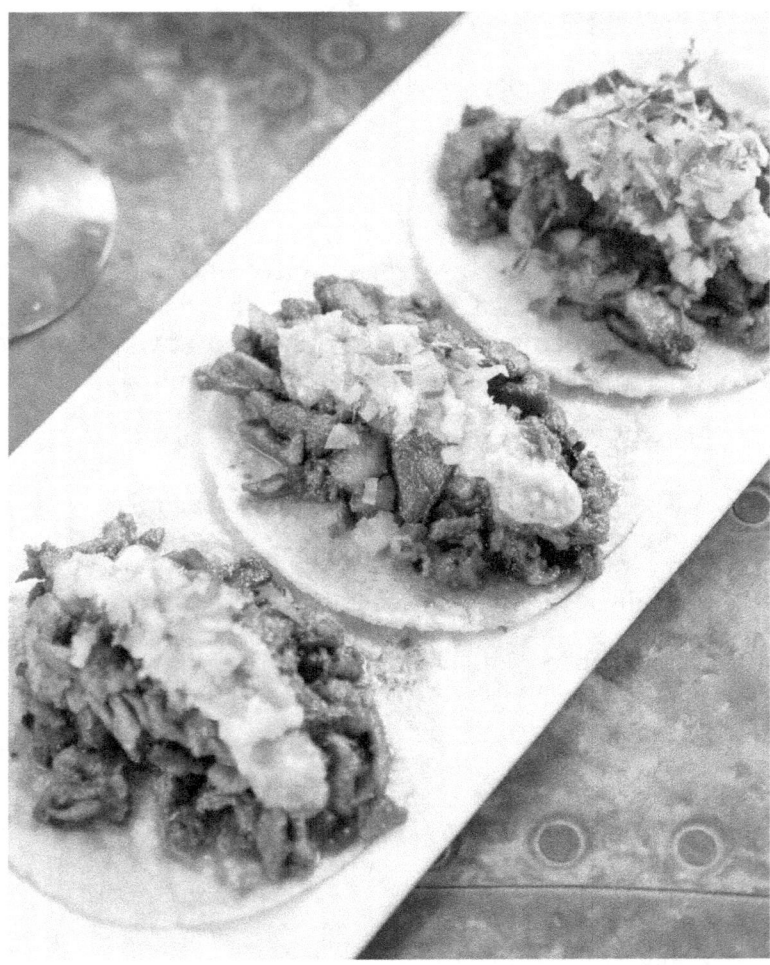

This recipe is hands down the best al pastor I have ever had, and I'm not just saying that because this is my recipe. I have tried al pastor from countless restaurants and taco stands. Al pastor is traditionally made on a trompo, a vertical rotisserie fired by propane or mesquite charcoal. Slices of marinated pork are stacked on a rod and slowly rotated to create a char on all sides. The meat is then sliced off of the trompo, allowing the underlying layers to be charred as well.

This cooking style has its roots in the Middle East and is similar to how shawarma is made. A Middle Eastern dish made of beef and lamb. In the early 1900s, Lebanese immigrants migrated to Mexico, and this cooking style was adapted to Mexican cuisine, and Al Pastor was born. Al pastor translates to "Shepard style," reflecting its origins from Shepard's in the Middle East.

Most of us don't have a trompo, so you must get creative to make this recipe at home. I made custom roasting rods using an extra oven rack. I cut a rod the rack, shaped a base out of one end, and sharpened the other end to make it easier to thread the meat onto it. You can use metal or wooden skewers if you don't have the time to make your own roasting rods. If you use wooden skewers, soak them in water so they don't burn. To use the skewer method, separate two skewers by a few inches to help hold up the stack of meat slices.

You can store your al pastor in the fridge for up to one week or up to 3 months in the freezer. If you freeze it in individual portions, you will have a quick meal anytime you crave some tacos.

This recipe requires you to marinate the meat for at least a few hours, but you can marinate it overnight for optimum results. The longer you marinate the meat, the more flavorful your dish will be.

I do not like much cumin, but you could add more to this recipe if you wish. If you're following a Carnivore or Keto diet, you could leave out the whole pineapple. Don't worry; you will still some pineapple flavor from the marinade.

This dish is customarily served as tacos with cilantro onion and topped with chile and freshly squeezed lemon. Chile is a Mexican hot sauce made with roasted tomatoes or tomatillos, roasted chili peppers, onions, garlic, and salt. These tacos go great with a side of radishes and sliced cucumbers.

Al pastor also makes for a fantastic filling for quesadillas, along with healthy amount of mozzarella cheese.

Difficulty Level: 4 out of 5 Meatballs

Prep Time: 20 Minutes

Cook Time: 1 1/2 Hours

Servings: 6

Nutritional Facts: (Per Serving)
Calories 416
Protein 45g
Fat 16g
Total Carbohydrates 19g

5 pounds of pork shoulder

1 pineapple, washed, peeled, and sliced into 1-inch rings

Marinade:

3 tablespoons of achiote paste

5 guajillo chilies, soaked in 2 cups of hot water until tender, stem and seeds removed

1 bulb of garlic, peeled and roughly chopped

1 tablespoon of oregano

1 tablespoon of cumin

1 tablespoon of salt

1 tablespoon of pepper

3/4 cup of apple cider vinegar

1 cup of pineapple juice

Slice the Pork into 1/4-inch thick slices and set aside.

Add all marinade ingredients into a zip-top bag or other container with a lid and stir to mix. Add the sliced pork, seal, and place in the fridge for 2-8 hours.

Remove the pork from the marinade and let it warm to room temperature.

Remove the middle rack from the oven and move the lower rack to the lowest slot, then preheat the oven to 350°F.

Thread one slice of pineapple onto the roasting rod, followed by a few slices of pork, and continue alternating threading the pineapple and pork onto the roasting rod and top with a piece of pineapple.

Place roasting rods on a baking sheet and bake at 350°F for 1 1/2 hours.

Remove from oven and let cool for 10 minutes.

Remove pork and pineapple from the roasting rod and chop into 1/2-inch pieces, making sure to discard the center portions of the pineapple. Mix the pineapple and pork together thoroughly.

In a large skillet over high heat, fry small batches of the pork and pineapple mixture until they get slightly charred.

Serve with onions and cilantro, and enjoy!

TURKEY

While the recipes in this cookbook focus on ground turkey, turkey as a whole can be prepared in many ways. From roasted turkey breasts to slow-cooked legs, there's no shortage of ways to prepare this bird. However, I've found that turkey tends to be relatively lean, which can leave some cuts a bit dry or lacking in flavor. That's why I prefer using ground turkey. It's easier to work with, more adaptable, and pairs beautifully with additional fat and other ingredients to create flavorful, satisfying dishes.

Ground turkey's mild flavor means it can take on a variety of seasonings, making it an excellent base for anything from burgers to meatballs to casseroles. In my recipes, you'll see I often add extra fats, such as cottage cheese or parmesan cheeses, along with herbs and spices. This improves the texture and enhances the depth of flavor, ensuring every bite is rich and enjoyable.

If you're feeling adventurous, I encourage you to explore other turkey preparations outside this chapter. Roasting a whole bird is always an option, and turkey thighs or wings can be braised for tender, juicy results. Whether you stick with ground turkey or branch out into other cuts, turkey is a great protein to experiment with in your kitchen and an excellent way to diversify your diet.

Turkey Nuggets

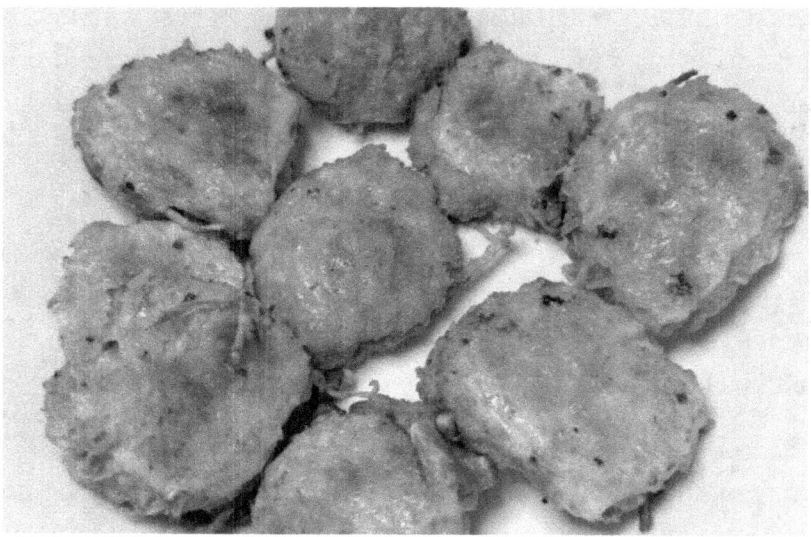

This ultra-low-carb take on traditional chicken nuggets is a recipe the whole family can get on board with. If you take the time to get them nice and crispy, kids and picky eaters will beg for more.

Chicken nuggets are traditionally breaded with flour, bread crumbs, and seasoning, then fried. They were invented in the United States around the 1950s and gained popularity in the 1980s with the introduction of the McDonalds chicken McNugget in 1983 and became a staple food item for kids and adults alike.

These nuggets are great with the accompanying cottage cheese-based ranch dip recipe, and they also go great with my no-sugar-added ketchup recipe found on page 51.

I have included directions for making them in an air fryer or baking them in an oven for your convenience.

When portioning the meat mixture, you can use a measuring spoon or a #30 disher (Ice cream scoop) to measure the mixture. One tip for making this step easier is to wet your spoon or disher with water between each scoop. Doing this will keep the meat mixture from sticking.

This recipe makes 36 nuggets, so you can adjust the proportions to make a smaller batch if you like, but these nuggets do freeze well and make for a wonderful last-minute meal. The best way to reheat them is in an air fryer or under a broiler to get them nice and crispy again. If you plan to store them, you don't have to get them super crispy when you first make them. You can do this when you reheat them.

The best part of this recipe is how crispy these nuggets get without deep frying them. If you're having trouble crisping them up, separate them into smaller batches and continue cooking them in an air fryer or under a broiler.

If you want more flavor, add taco seasoning to the pork rind mixture or add onion and garlic to the ground turkey mixture. This is a great opportunity to customize this recipe and make it your own. You could even add red pepper flakes for some heat.

Pork Panko

What is pork panko? It's ground pork rinds! These make a wonderful substitution for a binder or a crust, as per this recipe, and it's easy to make.

> Add pork rinds to a blender or food processor and process them until they form a flour-like consistency and no lumps are left.

You could skip the pork panko altogether for this recipe if you like, but they really help form a nice crust on the nuggets.

Difficulty Level: 3 out of 5 Meatballs

Prep Time: 20 Minutes

Cook Time: 16-30 Minutes

Servings: 6 (6 nuggets per serving)

Nutritional Facts:
(Per Serving)

Calories 563

Protein 79g

Fat 24g

Total Carbohydrates

3 eggs

3/4 cup cottage cheese

1 tablespoon of Worcestershire sauce

1 teaspoon of pepper

1 tablespoon of total seasoning

2 ½ pounds of ground turkey

2-3 cups parmesan cheese, shredded

6oz pork panko

Crack eggs into a large bowl and scramble with a fork. Add the cottage cheese, Worcestershire sauce, pepper, total seasoning, and only **1/3 cup** of the parmesan cheese into the bowl and mix.

Now, add the ground turkey into the bowl and mix until it is well combined and uniform consistency is achieved.

Cover the bowl and refrigerate it for at least one hour to allow it to firm up, making it easier to form the nuggets.

When you're ready to proceed, combine the pork rind crumbs and the remaining parmesan cheese in a medium bowl and set aside.

Preheat your cooking equipment of choice (see temperatures below).

Measure 2 tablespoons of the ground turkey mixture, roll it into a ball and place it in the pork panko mixture. Sprinkle some pork panko mixture on top and press it to form a 1/2-inch thick nugget. Make sure to coat the side of each nugget as well.

Shake off any excess pork panko mixture, place it on a parchment paper-lined baking sheet, and repeat this until all of the ground turkey mixture is used, placing the nuggets one inch apart from each other so they cook properly. You should be able to make approximately 36 nuggets.

Cooking your nuggets:

> **Oven**: Bake at 425°F for 20 minutes, then carefully turn each nugget over and continue baking for another 8-10 minutes or an internal temperature of 160°F is reached.

> **Air fryer**: Air fry at 450°F for 8 minutes. Carefully turn each nugget over and continue air frying for another 8 minutes or until an internal temperature of 160°F is reached.

To get your nuggets nice and crispy, take one serving at a time and either air fry at 450°F or place them under a broiler for 3-5 minutes.

Let the nuggets cool while you make the ranch dip, then chow down!

Ranch Dip

This recipe is a cottage cheese based ranch dip that can be adjusted to make ranch dressing. Substitute the ranch powder with onion dip mix to make a healthy onion dip. The sky is the limit for all the variations of this recipe.

By adjusting the amount of water you add, you can adapt this recipe to make a variety of sauces, dips, and dressings. The more water, the thinner it will be, which is ideal for dressings. The less water you add, the thicker it becomes, perfect for dips.

This recipe makes four servings and is best suited for a small smoothie or built-style blender. You can use a full-size blender if you are making a larger batch.

This dip stores well in the fridge for up to one week.

I also have an amazing blue cheese dip similar to this recipe, which goes great with steak and can be found on page 47.

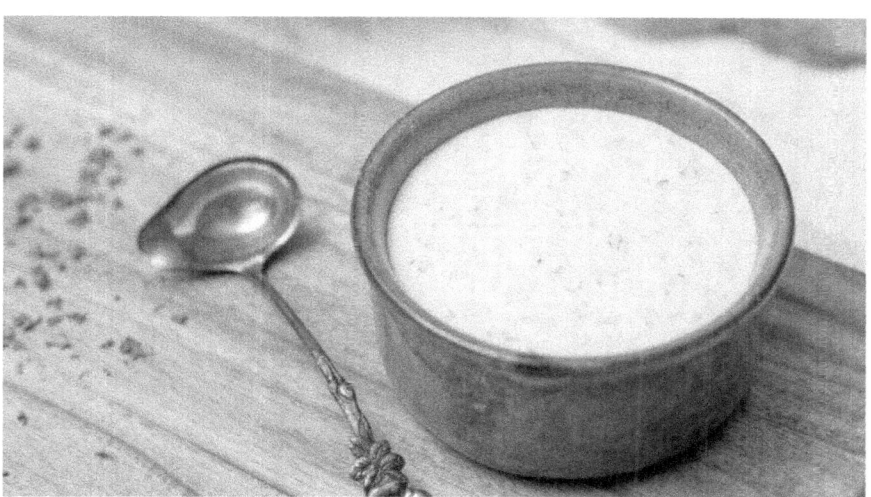

Difficulty Level: 1 out of 5 Meatballs

Prep Time: 2 Minutes

Cook Time: None

Servings: 4

> 1 cup of cottage cheese
>
> 2 tablespoons of filtered water
>
> 1 tablespoon ranch dip mix

Nutritional Facts:
(Per Serving)

Calories 61

Protein 5g

Fat 2g

Total Carbohydrates

Combine all of the ingredients in a blender.

Blend for approximately 1 minute or until smooth, scraping down the sides of the blender as needed.

Refrigerate for 20 minutes to thicken the dip and Enjoy!

Turkey Croquette Benedict

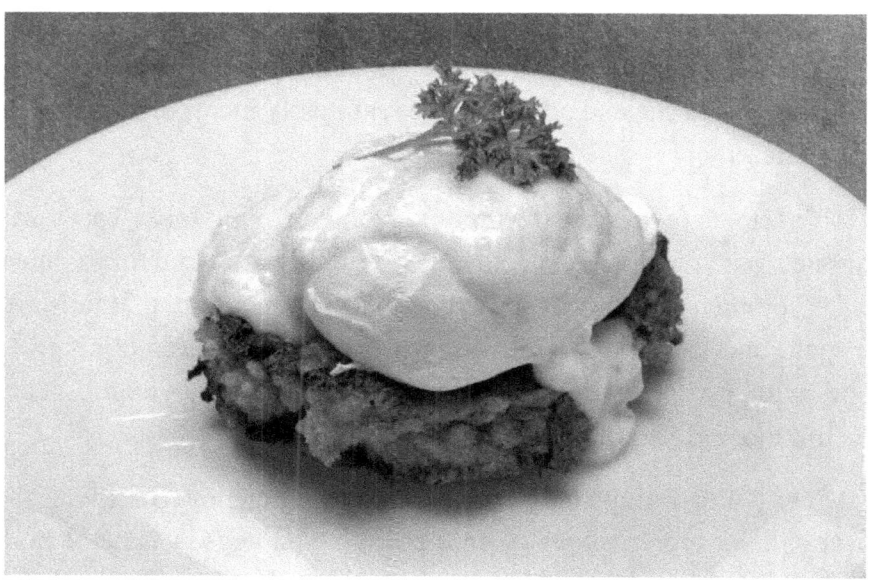

This recipe is the fanciest in this cookbook. It is a simple process, but several steps are involved. That is why I have rated it a four out of five on the meatball difficulty scale. However, if you prepare this recipe in advance and take your time, you will succeed in making this dish, even if you are new to cooking, and your friends and family will undoubtedly be impressed.

Croquettes come from French cuisine, their name comes from the French word croquer (to crunch). They are fried cylinders, balls, or patties of minced vegetables, seafood, or meat bound together by mashed potato or béchamel sauce. I have adapted and combined this recipe with Eggs Benedict to create a unique low-carbohydrate culinary experience.

Feel free to experiment by substituting the ground turkey with any other ground meat or seafood. You can also replace the parmesan cheese with your cheese of choice to create a distinctive flavor or substitute the parsley for another herb.

A food processor can be used to mince the garlic and onion, but this can also be done by hand without much difficulty. Sometimes, it's more work to clean the food processor than to mince by hand. However, if you end up mincing by hand, make sure to chop them into fine pieces. Use a box grater for the onion if you have one. If you do this right, the garlic and onion will be seamlessly incorporated into the croquette.

It's vital to refrigerate the mixture before cooking for at least thirty minutes, but you could refrigerate it overnight if preparing in advance, as I recommend for this dish. As the mixture warms up, that fat starts to melt, and the mixture will become mushy and extremely hard to work with, especially during dredging. For this reason, you must cool the mixture before frying.

Set up a dredging station for maximum efficiency. Start with the turkey mixture on one end, then the scrambled eggs, a plate of pork panko, and your stovetop with a frying pan ready to go. You will also want to have a baking sheet with a cooling rack or paper towels nearby to place the cooked croquettes so they don't get soggy after frying. Setting up your dredging station in this order will streamline the process so you can knock them out like a pro.

I recommend preparing the poached eggs and croquets in advance, but hollandaise sauce is best fresh, as it is hard to reheat without breaking the emulsion. You can store the cooked croquettes in the fridge for up to a week.

I have included my hollandaise sauce recipe following this recipe.

To serve the dish, place a croquette on a warm plate and place a fried or poached egg on top. See page 138 for my Perfectly Poached Egg recipe. Pour a portion of hollandaise sauce over the egg and garnish it with a sprig of parsley.

Difficulty Level: 4 out of 5 Meatballs

Prep Time: 20 Minutes

Cook Time: 8 Minutes

Servings: 4

Nutritional Facts:
(Per Serving)

Calories 330

Protein 40g

Fat 15g

Total Carbohydrates

1 pound of ground turkey

2 tablespoons of balsamic vinegar

1 tablespoon of Worcestershire sauce

1 teaspoon of salt

1/2 teaspoon of pepper

1 medium white onion, grated

1 garlic clove, minced fine

2 tablespoons of parsley, minced

1 tablespoons of sage, minced

1/2 cup buttermilk

2 eggs

1 cup of pork panko

2 tablespoons of clarified butter

Place all ingredients except 1 of the eggs and half of the pork panko in a medium-sized bowl and mix until well combined. Refrigerate for a minimum of 1 hour.

Prepare the hollandaise sauce and keep warm.

Divide the ground turkey mixture into 4 equal parts and form each portion into patties.

Scramble the reserved egg in a bowl wide enough to hold a patty and spread the reserved pork panko on a small plate. Set up your dredging station, starting with the patties, then the egg, and finally the pork panko.

Place a skillet over medium-high heat and add a tablespoon of the clarified butter. When the skillet is hot but not burning, dip one of the patties into the egg and then the pork panko. Flip the patty over to cover the other side in pork panko and place it in the hot skillet.

Cook for 1 minute on each side or until cooked all the way through. Place on a paper towel and continue this process with the remaining patties.

To serve, place your croquette on a warmed plate, place a poached egg on top of the croquette, cover with a portion of hollandaise sauce, garnish with parsley, and enjoy!

Hollandaise Sauce

Hollandaise sauce is a thick, creamy, yellow sauce made from egg yolks and butter and flavored with lemon juice. It is one of the most well-known sauces in French cooking and can be modified for various dishes.

This traditional hollandaise sauce recipe is decadent and delicious; if you follow the directions closely, you will find success with this recipe.

If your butter is too hot, it will scramble the egg. If you add the butter too fast, your sauce may not come together, and the end product will be granular. This is why you must pour the melted butter as slowly as possible; drop by drop is an excellent place to start, especially at the beginning. Getting your butter to as close to two hundred degrees Fahrenheit as possible will slowly cook the yolk without overcooking them.

To properly separate the egg yolk from the white, set out two bowls. Then gently crack an egg over the first bowl and separate the shell into two halves, letting the egg whites fall into the bowl. Transfer the yolk between the shells until all or most of the whites have been removed. Finally, place the yolk into the second bowl. Repeat this process with the rest of the eggs. Do not discard the reserved egg whites. They can be used for many other recipes.

Using a blender, food processor, or an emersion blender will make producing this recipe much easier, but you can do it by hand if that's all you have. Well, you'll need a whisk, but I digress. If using a food processor or an emersion blender, follow the recipe as usual.

If making by hand, use a small saucepan over the lowest setting on your stove, and instead of blending, use your whisk to incorporate the butter. If your pan gets too hot, cool it off by placing it in cool water and then back to the stove.

Once you have added about half of the butter, the sauce should be thick and creamy. If it separates, you can try removing the sauce from the blender and, with the blender on high speed, add the mixture back in very slowly. This technique may save your sauce. If not, start over. If you take your time, you will get it, and trust me, this sauce is worth it.

Customize this recipe by adding fresh herbs or a dash of your favorite hot sauce. You can even add tomato paste to create a Choron sauce that is great for meat and egg dishes. You can do so much with such basic ingredients and your imagination. This is one of the many reasons I love cooking. You can make it your own and experiment to find what you like best.

With this recipe, you can also make a Béarnaise sauce by replacing the lemon juice with a reduction of wine vinegar, dry white wine, shallots, and tarragon. This goes great on steaks!

This recipe is best served fresh but can be stored in the fridge for about three days. You must be very careful not to break the sauce when reheating. The best way to do this is to use a microwave on the lowest setting for fifteen seconds, followed by fifteen seconds of rest. Mix and test the temperature and repeat as needed.

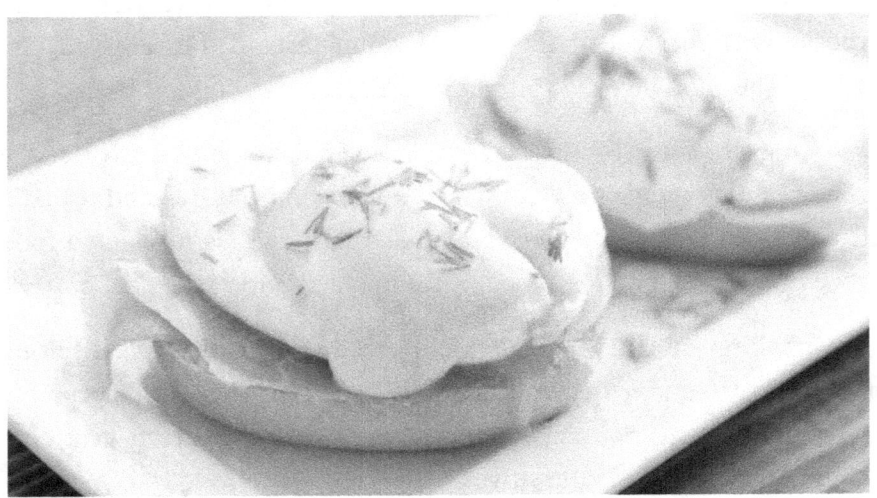

Hollandaise sauce tastes great on burger patties, steak, and on my pork panko crusted chicken found on page 104.

Difficulty Level: 3 out of 5 Meatballs

Prep Time: 10 Minutes

Cook Time: 2-5 Minutes

Servings: 4

Nutritional Facts:
(Per Serving)

Calories 272

Protein 2g

Fat 29g

Total Carbohydrates > 1g

4.5 ounces of butter

3 egg yolks

1 teaspoon of lemon juice

1/4 teaspoon of salt

A pinch of pepper

Melt the butter in a microwave or in a saucepan on the stove. It needs to be close to 200°F.

Add the egg yolks, salt, pepper, and lemon juice in a blender pitcher. Cover and blend at high speed for a few seconds.

With the blender still on, remove the lid and slowly pour the melted butter into the egg yolk mixture. You can discard the white milk solids that accumulate underneath the butter.

Taste and adjust seasoning as needed. Then, serve immediately or keep it in a warm place if made in advance.

Ultra Low-Carb Turkey Fries

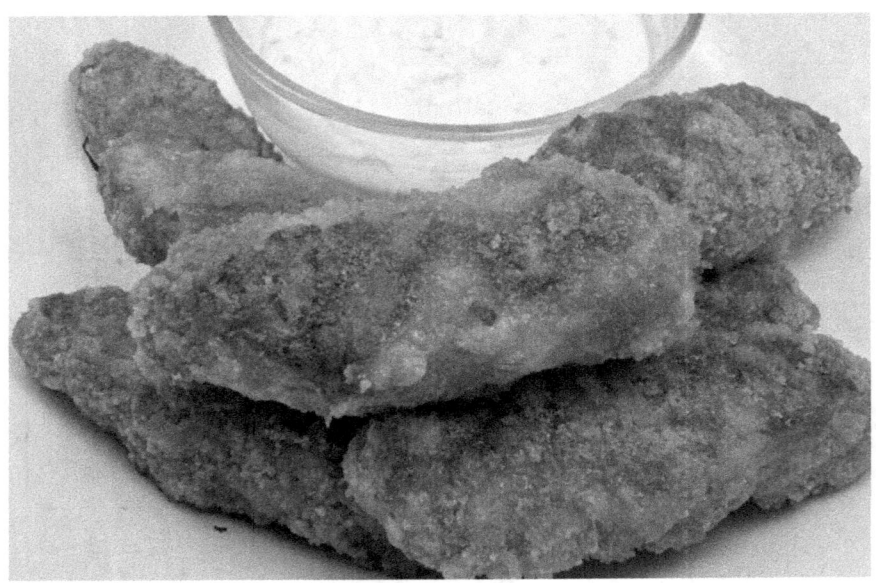

Fast-food chicken fries don't have ish on these ultra-low-carb turkey fries! I love to eat these fries with my Ranch Dip recipe found on page 159. I have also provided detailed instructions on preparing pork panko, a zero-carb breading made from pork rinds, on page 156.

A baking rack, also known as a cooling rack, will take your fries to the next level. However, it's all good if you don't have one. After baking, you can throw the fries under a broiler or in an air fryer to get them to crisp-fection.

Forming the fries for the first time can be a bit intimidating, but no worries; you will get the hang of it. Start by measuring out two tablespoons of the ground turkey mixture, then use your hands to form it into a ball. Then, roll the ball between your hands to form a cylinder. Use the width of your hand as a frame of reference for the length of each fry. You may need to push the ends slightly to get a uniform shape.

If you're running low on time, you can use this same mixture to make turkey patties by dividing the turkey mixture into four parts, forming them into patties, coat with panko, and bake at 350°F for 20 minutes.

It is essential to keep the ground turkey in the fridge until just before you make this recipe, as working with cold ground meat is much easier. When ground meat warms up, the fat softens, making it harder to work with. This is also why you must freeze the fries for twenty minutes before coating them with the pork panko.

When the fries are done, they should be golden brown; they will become crispy once they cool a bit. If they do not crisp up to your expectations, place one serving in an air fryer at four hundred degrees Fahrenheit for five minutes or broil on the top shelf of your oven for three to five minutes. If your fries are too crowded, they will not get crispy, so give them space.

You can freeze your fries before or after you bake them for up to three months. If you freeze them raw, you will need to bread them in the pork panko before they thaw completely and bake as stated in the instructions. Baked fries will last in the fridge for up to a week.

Feel free to substitute or add additional seasonings per your preferences. If you want to add heat, try including red pepper flakes or more paprika.

This recipe was inspired by a healthy chicken nugget recipe I found online and has been adapted to meet my standards of flavor and nutrition.

Difficulty Level: 3 out of 5 Meatballs

Prep Time: 10 Minutes

Cook Time: 20 Minutes

Servings: 2

Nutritional Facts: (Per Serving)
Calories 427
Protein 69g
Fat 15g
Total Carbohydrates

1 pound of ground turkey

1 egg

1/2 cup of shredded parmesan cheese

1/2 teaspoon of garlic powder

1/2 teaspoon of onion powder

1/4 teaspoon of smoked paprika

1 teaspoon of salt

1/4 teaspoon of pepper

1/2 cup pork panko

Mix the ground turkey, egg, parmesan cheese, and seasonings together in a medium-sized bowl until well combined.

Roll 2 tablespoons of the meat mixture in your hands to form a ball, then move your hands back and forth with light pressure to create a cylindrical shape. Use the width of your hand as a gauge for the length of the fry. Make them as uniform as possible; makes 16 fries.

Place fries on a parchment paper lined baking sheet and place in the freezer for 20 minutes.

Preheat oven to 450°F.

Remove from the freezer, place the pork panko on a plate or wide bottom bowl, and roll each of the fries in the pork panko. Cover the ends and tap the fry on the side of the bowl to remove any excess breading.

Place a baking rack on top of a baking sheet and evenly space the fries on the rack.

Bake at 450°F for 9 minutes, flip each fry over, and bake for another 9 minutes or until they reach an internal temperature of 160°F.

If the fries are not crispy, remove half of them, place them on the top rack of your oven, and broil on high heat for 3-5 minutes.

Let cool on the baking rack for 5 min so they can crisp up and enjoy!

WHEY PROTEIN POWDER

Whey protein powder isn't something I recommend as a primary protein source, but it can be a fantastic tool to help you meet your protein goals, especially when you're beginning to increase your protein intake. If you're working on building muscle or losing fat, adding whey protein powder into smoothies, snacks, and sweet treats makes it easier to stay on track.

Whey protein is fast-digesting, which makes it an ideal option post-workout, helping your muscles recover quickly. It can also be used in many applications and is a seamless way to sneak extra protein into meals without much effort.

In this chapter, you'll find recipes that creatively incorporate whey protein. These recipes are designed to provide flavor and nutrition in one package, helping you stay satisfied.

Although whey protein is useful, I believe in focusing on whole food proteins whenever possible—foods like eggs, meat, and dairy offer more complete nutrient profiles and should form the foundation of your diet. But when time is tight or you need an extra boost, whey protein powder can be a great ally. Use it wisely, experiment with these recipes, and enjoy its convenience.

Chocolate Peanut Butter Protein Bars

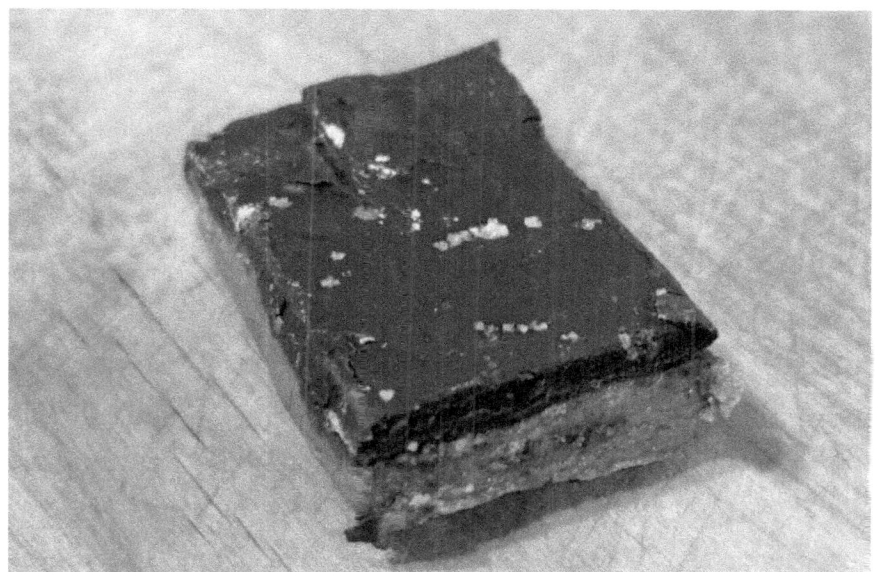

Only make these if you have company coming over because these chocolate peanut butter protein bars are so good you will want to eat them all. You can also make a smaller portion if you have poor self-control with sweets like I do. These taste better than Reese's peanut butter cups, and each bar has 14 grams of protein!

To save time during cleanup, use a 2-cup or bigger measuring cup to measure the peanut butter, then add the maple syrup and mix. Then, mix the protein powder until all ingredients are well incorporated. It should have a consistency similar to cookie dough. If the nougat mixture is too sticky, add more protein powder.

I keep my peanut butter in the fridge because I use natural peanut butter that only contains peanuts and salt. I have found that this practice helps the nougat to be more solid. Try refrigerating your peanut butter or the nougat itself if it is too soft.

When you form the peanut butter nougat layer in the pan, it can be tricky to get it evenly distributed due to its thickness. One trick is to press on a piece of parchment paper on top of the nougat to form a uniform layer. If you have another pan that fits inside the first pan, press it down on the parchment paper to form the nougat into an even layer.

If you don't have a 4x8-inch pan, you can use another size pan. However, this may affect the thickness of the nougat layer and change the ratio of nougat to chocolate. You can also use silicone muffin liners to make peanut butter protein cups, but you will need to use more chocolate to have enough for each cup.

When melting the chocolate chips and the coconut oil, make sure to microwave them only for 20 seconds at a time, then stir to help it melt faster and repeat as needed. Once the chocolate chips and the coconut oil are melted, pour the melted chocolate mixture directly on top of the nougat layer.

Once the chocolate has solidified in the fridge, you can cut it into bars directly on the parchment paper. If you divide this recipe into twelve bars, two bars would equal one serving.

Your chocolate peanut butter protein bars can be stored on the parchment paper in a sealed container in the fridge for up to one week or frozen for up to six months.

I originally discovered this recipe online and adapted it to make it my own. You can make it your own by experimenting with milk chocolate chips instead of dark chocolate chips, but I recommend dark chocolate as it has less sugar. You can also try replacing the maple syrup with honey or add some vanilla extract. I have also found that vanilla-flavored protein powder works well.

A chocolate chip peanut butter cookie dough can also be made from this recipe by adding the chocolate chips directly into the nougat mixture and mix them in, then roll the mixture into a log and cut it into slices.

Difficulty Level: 2 out of 5 Meatballs

Prep Time: 5 Minutes

Cook Time: 1 Minute

Servings: 6

Nutritional Facts:
(Per Serving)

Calories 359

Protein 14g

Fat 27g

Total Carbohydrates 17g

1 cup of peanut butter

1 tablespoon of maple syrup

1 scoop of whey protein powder
(chocolate or vanilla flavored)

1/3 cup (2.5 ounces) of dark chocolate chips

1 tablespoon of coconut oil

1 teaspoon of coarse sea salt

In a small bowl, combine the peanut butter and the maple syrup and mix until well combined. Add in the protein powder and mix until fully incorporated and a thick nougat is formed.

Place the nougat mixture into an 8x4-inch pan lined with parchment paper. Use another piece of parchment paper and your hands to level out the nougat layer.

In a small microwave-safe bowl, combine the chocolate chips and the coconut oil, microwave for 20 seconds, stir, and repeat until the chocolate is fully melted.

Pour the melted chocolate mixture over the peanut butter nougat. Spread the chocolate mixture by tilting the pan from side to side in alternating directions, then lightly tap the pan on your countertop to help distribute the chocolate mixture evenly.

Place in the fridge for 10 minutes, sprinkle the sea salt on the chocolate, and place in the freezer for 1 hour. Cut into 12 bars and try not to eat them all.

Stacked Peanut Butter Protein Shake

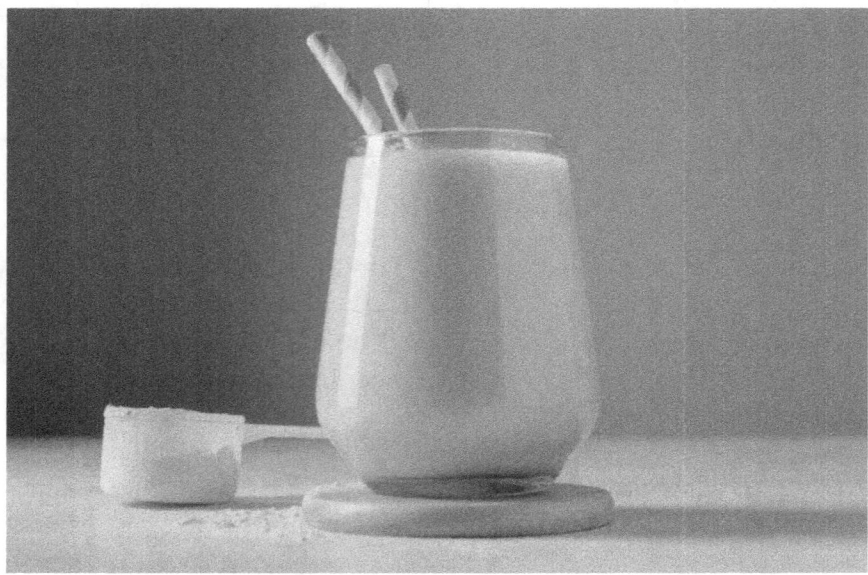

This protein shake is great for a post-workout meal that will maximize your recovery or anytime you need extra protein. It packs a whopping fifty grams of protein at only 315 calories, and it tastes so good you will want to drink it daily!

I love the flavor that the coconut water adds, in addition to the added electrolytes in the form of potassium and sodium. You can use water instead of coconut water in a pinch. Choose a brand of coconut water with no added sugar and is not made from concentrate.

If you're looking to bulk up, use whole raw milk instead of coconut water. Milk is calorie-dense and provides many nutrients to support your overall health and muscle growth.

Pro tip: Your shakes will taste much better if your liquid of choice is cold.

I use Gold Standard 100% Whey Protein Isolate Powder, and I like the Vanilla Ice Cream flavor because it tastes amazing. A Chocolate or even an unflavored whey protein isolate powder would also work well for this recipe. I know Gold Standard is not the highest quality whey protein isolate powder, but it is economical and widely available. If you want a cleaner nose-to-tail protein powder that includes colostrum, beef organs, and is whey-free, try using noble origin all-in-one protein powder. I love the chocolate flavor because it tastes amazing (No hint of organ meats) and is easy to digest. If you use this, you can skip the collagen peptides because they are already in this protein powder.

Peanut butter powder adds flavor, additional protein, and slows down the absorption of the protein due to the fat and fiber it contains. These nutrients are digested slower than protein, and when you combine them, it leads to slower absorption, keeping you feeling fuller for longer and also helps your body absorb more of that vital protein. Peanut butter powder has fewer calories and fat than traditional peanut butter, it's portable, and you don't need to use a blender to make your shake as you would with traditional peanut butter. I use the Original PB Fit Peanut Butter powder.

I have included collagen peptides in this recipe to increase the protein and its other health benefits to your skin, joints, bones, gut, hair, and nails.

Fiber is an integral part of a healthy diet because it will slow down absorption and keep you feeling fuller for longer. Eating a high-protein diet can make it hard to get fiber, so I included psyllium husk powder in this recipe. Make sure to drink your shake soon after you make it, or it will become very thick due to the psyllium husk powder.

I also add five grams of creatine monohydrate to my shakes for all of the many health benefits it provides. Creatine is one of the most studied supplements out there. It has been shown to help build muscle mass, increase strength gains, help avoid fatigue, make your bones stronger, improve brain health, and can even assist in overcoming depression. Other positive benefits include anti-inflammatory properties and shortened muscle recovery time.

I use a blender bottle when I make this recipe because it is portable and easy to use. It is a bottle with a wire ball that helps mix the ingredients and has a spout so you can drink your shake directly from it.

If you want to save time, you can mix up a few batches of the dry ingredients in separate containers. Then, when you are ready for a shake, all you have to do is dump the pre-measured dry ingredients into your blender bottle, add the coconut water, shake to mix, and chug it down!

Protein shakes are a great tool for adding more protein to your diet or when you are short on time, but I don't recommend using them as a primary source of protein because the protein is highly processed. Your body will get so much more from whole unprocessed animal protein.

Difficulty Level: 1 out of 5 Meatballs

Prep Time: 3 Minutes

Cook Time: None

Servings: 1

Nutritional Facts:
(Per Serving)

Calories 315

Protein 50g

Fat 3.5g

Total Carbohydrates 25g

11 fluid ounces of organic coconut water

1 scoop (31g) protein powder (vanilla or chocolate)

2 tablespoons of peanut butter powder

4 tablespoons of collagen peptides

1 teaspoon of psyllium husk powder

1 scoop (5 grams) of creatine monohydrate

Combine all of the dry ingredients in a blender bottle.

Pour the coconut water into the bottle, screw on the lid, and make sure the spout cap is closed.

Shake vigorously until all ingredients are well incorporated and there are no lumps.

Drink and enjoy the many benefits this protein shake provides!

Blueberry and Chia Seed Pudding

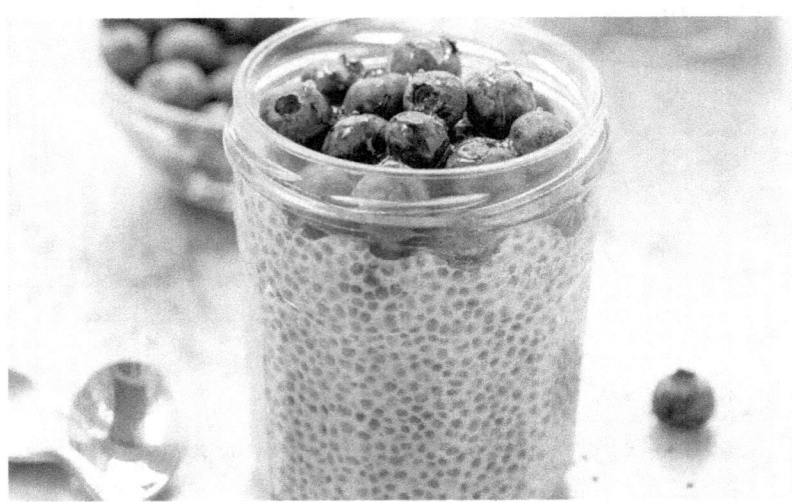

This recipe is a great snack and ideal for meal prep. The only thing that sucks about this recipe is that you have to wait for the chia seeds to absorb the coconut water before you can eat it, don't fret; it takes less than an hour in the fridge for this to take place, and you are left with a thick and delicious pudding.

Coconut water adds sweetness and electrolytes to this dish. You could use water instead, but if you have coconut water, use it. You'll thank me after you try it. I recommend using coconut water with no added sugar.

Once the pudding is prepared, it will be runny, but don't worry— the chia seeds are the key to the lovely consistency of this recipe. Once they absorb the coconut water, the pudding will thicken up, and the additional soluble fiber from the seeds will help you stay regular.

The purpose of the kefir is to incorporate additional probiotics to this recipe to help your gut function properly.

I like to prepare this snack in advance using six half-pint wide-mouth mason jars. These are convenient to grab out of the fridge and take with you when you need a refreshing snack on the go.

Start by adding the coconut water, Greek yogurt, and protein powder to a medium-sized bowl and mix until well combined. Line up the mason jars and add half a cup of the yogurt mixture to each jar. The extra bit can be used to make a smaller portion of pudding right in the yogurt container. Now add one-quarter cup of coconut water, one tablespoon of chia seeds, one tablespoon of Kiefer, and a couple of blueberries to each jar. Now for the fun part! Close each jar and shake vigorously to mix everything. Then refrigerate them for at least one hour, and you're all set.

This pudding will store in the fridge for up to one week. You can substitute the vanilla protein powder for a chocolate-flavored protein powder for a more dessert-like snack, if you do this I would not add the blueberries. If you choose to not add the protein powder, I recommend using a vanilla-flavored yogurt or adding some vanilla extract. You can also replace the blueberries with your berry of choice, or peaches would also work well in this dish.

This recipe was inspired by an overnight oat recipe my wife used to make. I wanted something that was easy to grab out of the fridge, refreshing, and low-carb, and this recipe is the result of that.

Difficulty Level: 1 out of 5 Meatballs

Prep Time: 5 Minutes

Cook Time: None

Servings: 4

Nutritional Facts:
(Per Serving)

Calories 210

Protein 24g

Fat 4g

Total Carbohydrates 14g

2 cups of Greek yogurt

2 scoops of vanilla protein powder

1 cup of coconut water

4 tablespoons of chia seeds

4 tablespoons of goat milk kefir

1/2 cup of blueberries

Mix the Greek yogurt and protein powder until well combined in a medium-sized bowl.

Add the coconut water, kefir, and chia seeds into the yogurt mixture and mix well.

Fold the blueberries into the mixture, cover, and refrigerate for at least one hour, then enjoy!

Note From the Author:

Thank you for joining me on this journey to better health, strength, and vitality. Writing *The Protein Lifestyle Cookbook* has been a labor of love, and knowing that you've taken the time to explore these recipes means the world to me.

This book was born out of a passion for creating sustainable, protein-forward habits that fuel the body and mind. I hope these recipes have nourished you and inspired you to take control of your health in a way that feels empowering and achievable.

To those of you who've experimented, adapted, and made these dishes your own—bravo! Cooking isn't about perfection; it's about showing up for yourself and your loved ones with care and intention. Every time you plate up a meal, you build a stronger foundation for your future, one bite at a time.

If this cookbook has brought value to your life, I'd love to hear about your experience. Whether it's a favorite recipe, a newfound confidence in the kitchen, or a success story about your health journey, please don't hesitate to share it with me. You can reach me through JoshNoland.com.

Finally, remember that the protein lifestyle isn't about a single destination—it's a lifelong practice of growth, balance, and resilience. Stay curious, keep experimenting, and most importantly, be kind to yourself along the way.

With gratitude,

Joshua D. Noland

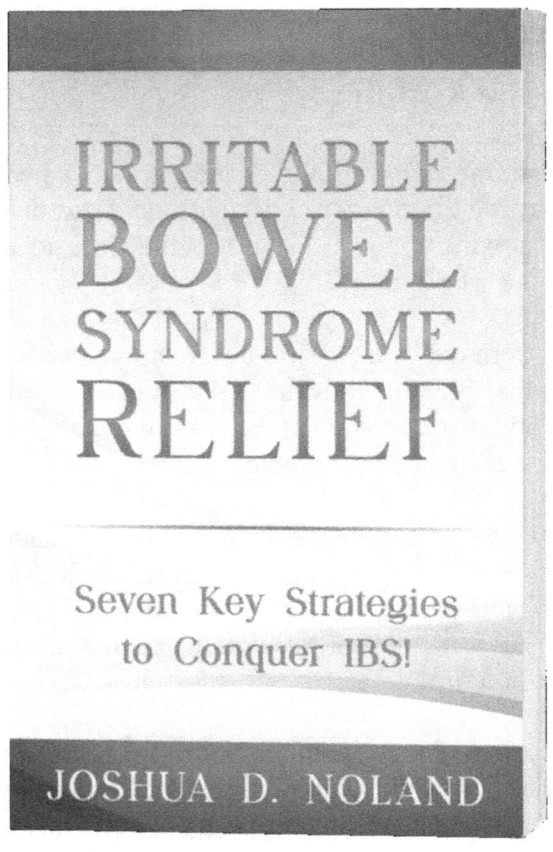

Are you newly diagnosed with Irritable Bowel Syndrome, a long-time sufferer seeking new solutions, or dealing with other digestive issues? This book is your comprehensive guide to naturally healing from IBS and preventing future flare-ups. Joshua D. Noland and countless others overcame IBS by following the tips and strategies outlined in this book. It takes a holistic approach, providing you with the tools to understand and manage your symptoms so you can start enjoying life again. By applying the knowledge you will gain in this book, you can reduce IBS symptoms, experience fewer flare-ups, and gain an improved quality of life.

IBS-Book.com

"When in doubt, add protein."

www.ingramcontent.com/pod-product-compliance
Lightning Source LLC
Chambersburg PA
CBHW080956120626
46546CB00010B/2915